Solve Your Food Intolerance

A practical dietary programme to eliminate food intolerance

Dr John Hunter

with Elizabeth Workman
and Jenny Woolner

LONDON

The authors wish to thank Mrs Pamela Harris for her invaluable help in designing many of the recipes.

7 9 10 8

This fifth edition published in 2005 by Vermilion, an imprint of Ebury Publishing
A Random House Group company

First published in the United Kingdom as *The New Allergy Diet* by Martin Dunitz Ltd in 1984
Second edition published by Macdonald Optima in 1988
Third edition published by Vermilion in 1996
Fourth edition published by Vermilion in 2000

The Random House Group Limited Reg. No. 954009

Addresses for companies within the Random House Group can be found at:
www.randomhouse.co.uk

A CIP catalogue record for this book is available from the British Library

ISBN 978-0-09-190665-8

To buy books by your favourite authors and register for offers visit:
www.randomhouse.co.uk

Although every effort has been made to ensure that the contents of this book
are accurate, it must not be treated as a substitute for qualified medical advice.
Neither the Author nor the Publisher can be held responsible for any loss or
claim arising out of the use, or misuse, of the suggestions made or the failure to
take medical advice.

The Random House Group Limited supports The Forest Stewardship
Council® (FSC®), the leading international forest-certification organisation.
Our books carrying the FSC label are printed on FSC®-certified paper.
FSC is the only forest-certification scheme supported by the leading
environmental organisations, including Greenpeace. Our
paper procurement policy can be found at
www.randomhouse.co.uk/environment

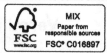

MIX
Paper from
responsible sources
FSC® C016897

Printed and bound in Great Britain by Clays Ltd, St Ives PLC

Contents

About the authors

John Hunter is a Consultant Physician at Addenbrooke's Hospital, Cambridge and a recognised authority on the subject of food allergy and intolerance. He developed an interest in food in relation to diseases of the gut as a result of the need of the many sufferers of irritable bowel syndrome attending his outpatients' clinic. He has contributed over a hundred research papers to major medical journals including *The Lancet, Nature* and the *British Medical Journal*.

Elizabeth Workman gained her State Registration as a dietitian after following the dietetics course at Leeds Metropolitan University, already being a holder of a Biological Sciences degree from Leicester University. She has gained great expertise in helping people with food-related diseases and enjoys the challenge of devising appetising and nutritious recipes from unusual ingredients.

Jenny Woolner graduated from Southampton University with a degree in Biochemistry and Physiology with nutrition, and obtained her State Registration as a dietitian and an MSC in Health Sciences from Leeds Metropolitan University. She has worked as a research dietitian with Dr Hunter for nine years, contributing to a number of research papers, combining this with bringing up her young family.

Introduction

Although most foods we eat are perfectly safe and healthy, sometimes people suffer unpleasant reactions after meals. Food poisoning is well understood; foods may contain bacteria that cause gastroenteritis. Spoiled food may contain chemicals that upset us – for example, if raw mackerel is allowed to become warm, histamine may be produced and this can cause diarrhoea and vomiting. Some people, however, may suffer unpleasant reactions after eating foods that are not contaminated in any way. A wide variety of symptoms may arise, such as headache, skin rashes and diarrhoea, and in some cases these become chronic problems that require deeper investigation. This book is dedicated to helping people decide if they may have such problems with foods and, if so, which foods are producing their symptoms.

There are several different ways in which foods may cause trouble, and these will be discussed in detail later in the book. It has been the custom for all unpleasant reactions to be termed as 'food allergies' but in reality relatively few are due to a genuine allergy. More commonly, these reactions may be caused by certain bacteria living in the gut, enzyme deficiencies, or simply the effects of chemicals that may be present in the food. We use the term 'food intolerance' because it does not presuppose the way in which the food has its effect, in order to cover all these possibilities.

As mechanisms of food intolerance vary greatly, there is no single test that will detect them. In many cases, diagnosis depends on the time-honoured methods of excluding and reintroducing foods in the diet to assess what effects they produce. This can prove a complicated and confusing business. Currently, few doctors have experience in this field, but in this book we set out the guidelines for detecting your food intolerances, and give advice on how best to cope with them.

What are allergies?

Most of the books written about food and disease call the condition 'food allergy'. Originally the word allergy meant an unpleasant reaction to any foreign substance in the body, but over the years it has changed, and now doctors use it to describe a reaction caused by a breakdown of the immune system.

The real job of the immune system is to recognize and destroy infecting agents such as bacteria and viruses that have got into the body. Substances in the blood called antibodies are produced and these make the cells defending the body attack the germs. In allergic reactions an abnormal type of antibody is produced that reacts to certain foreign substances called allergens, such as spores, pollens and foods. The combination of these antibodies with the allergen produces the allergic symptoms.

In most allergies doctors can detect the allergic reaction going on in the blood, but in the case of food intolerance this type of reaction is hardly ever found. This is why doctors have doubted the existence of such a condition as food allergy. Yet some foods have been proved to cause diseases.

How do foods cause diseases?

In some cases the role food plays in causing disease is well established. For example, coeliac disease is a condition in which gluten, a protein found in wheat, rye and barley, damages the lining of the small intestine so that food is not properly absorbed. This leads to a number of difficulties including diarrhoea, bone disease and failure to grow, or loss of weight. Anaemia may also result from these problems. Because the symptoms can be caused by several other conditions it is not safe to start a gluten-free diet as treatment without being diagnosed first by a specialist.

Coeliac disease is thought to affect about one in three hundred to one in two thousand people in the UK. The discovery that coeliac disease was caused by gluten was purely accidental. Most of the wheat grown in Holland during the Second World War was directed to the German army at the Front, so the civilian population had to make do with potatoes. At this time children with coeliac disease made dramatic improvements, and the Dutch specialist Dr W.K. Dicke made the connection that excluding gluten from the diet had made the children better.

People with coeliac disease recover completely once they avoid foods containing gluten. However, they should still be seen regularly by their specialist to make sure they are well and not lapsing on the diet, even by mistake.

Commercial gluten-free products are available on prescription to people with coeliac disease. Many of the recipes in this book are suitable for coeliacs and further help may be obtained from the Coeliac Society.

Another condition in which there is a link between food and symptoms is lactose intolerance. Lactose is a sugar contained in milk, which is digested by a natural chemical called an enzyme, found in the wall of the intestine. All children have this enzyme. It normally disappears in early adult life in African, Black American and Asian populations, and occasionally in Europeans. This means that some people may develop diarrhoea if they drink milk, because they are unable to break down the lactose.

Other foods contain chemicals that can upset some people. This may be linked to the way the various enzymes in their bodies behave. A clue in the discovery was the action of one of the enzymes called mono-amine oxidase. Certain drugs reduce its activity, and people who are taking them have to avoid eating foods such as cheese, red wine, yeast or yeast extract, otherwise they get high blood pressure and severe headaches.

Unfortunately, it is not always as simple as that; food intolerance is not always the result of the behaviour of enzymes. There are other chemicals that work in different ways, including caffeine, histamine and tyramine. Caffeine is found in tea, coffee, cocoa, cola drinks and chocolate; histamine in cheese, beer, sausages and some canned foods; and tyramine in brewer's yeast, red wine and cheese. Too much strong coffee produces many familiar symptoms: restlessness, palpitations and heartburn. Histamine and tyramine may be a cause of migraine. It is thought that when they are absorbed into the body they may change the diameter of small blood vessels, and so bring on an attack in people who get migraine.

In our research in Cambridge we have studied food intolerance in the irritable bowel syndrome in great detail. People often develop IBS (see below) after a bout of gastroenteritis, or repeated courses of antibiotics. Indeed, a recent study showed that as many as one-third of patients developing gastroenteritis went on to suffer long-term symptoms of IBS. In our experience, many patients with this condition demonstrate changes in the bacteria living in their intestines. It seems possible that these bacteria are responsible for the breakdown of food chemicals which cause IBS.

We tested this theory by studying the excretion of hydrogen and methane in patients with IBS. These chemicals can be produced in the human body only by the action of bowel bacteria. We found that, compared to healthy people, IBS patients produced large volumes of hydrogen and little or no methane. When we put them on the exclusion diet (discussed later in this book), this excess gas production fell to normal and symptoms cleared. Thus food intolerance in many cases of IBS is caused not by any allergy, but by abnormal fermentation in the large intestine.

As there are so many different causes of reactions to food,

and as most of them are nothing to do with allergy, you will see why we prefer to speak of 'food intolerance' rather than 'food allergy'.

Conditions caused by food intolerance

As we have explained, from the present state of knowledge about how foods cause disease, it cannot be said that food intolerance is the cause in every case. There are certainly other known causes for many of these conditions, but we and other researchers have shown by the success of our dietary treatment that food intolerance is one of the most common. If you or your child are diagnosed as having one of the conditions below, a special diet might be the remedy, but you must discuss this with your doctor and, if necessary, your specialist, before you start excluding foods from your daily intake.

The conditions listed below are the ones that may be caused by food intolerance and are therefore potentially treatable by diet. These are discussed in more detail in the next pages and suggestions are given as to the appropriate diets to try.

Irritable Bowel Syndrome	Migraine
Asthma	Eczema
Urticaria	Rhinitis
Some types of arthritis	Cow's milk sensitive
Hyperactivity and autism	enteropathy
in children	Crohn's disease

Irritable bowel syndrome

Irritable bowel syndrome is a very common condition that may affect as many as 8–22 per cent of the population at some time in their lives. Sufferers get abdominal pain and bloating, together with an upset in their bowel habit – diarrhoea or constipation. It accounts for 20–50 per cent of referrals to gastroenterology clinics in the developed world.

Repeated investigations such as x-rays and blood tests reveal no damage to the gut, leading doctors to believe that the condition is largely psychological. Treatment is often very unsatisfactory. This is usually because irritable bowel syndrome is not one single condition, but a collection of quite separate problems producing similar symptoms. In our experience approximately 20 per cent of cases are due to anxiety. The majority, however, are caused by food intolerance. Of the first 182 patients we treated by diet, we were able to relieve symptoms completely in 122. We wrote to 80 patients two years later to ask them how they were getting on and 71 replied: 59 were feeling well on their diets, six were still well and had gone back to normal eating, and only six had relapsed.

Although not all cases are caused by food intolerance – menstrual changes, too much or not enough fibre in the diet, or short-term stress can bring on symptoms – we believe that anyone with irritable bowel syndrome should at least try an exclusion diet. The use of diet in irritable bowel is explained in detail in the following chapter.

Migraine

Migraine is a very common problem. It is estimated that over five million people in England alone suffer from this illness. At least 90 per cent of people with migraine have attacks before the age of 40; most have their first attack during their teens or early twenties. In women there is a strong hereditary tendency and often a connection with the menstrual cycle. In some people the attacks develop quickly and last a few hours. In others they may be more drawn out, lasting one to three days. The headache is not always the main symptom of migraine and for many people nausea and vomiting are the major problems. Others also experience disturbed vision and flashing lights.

There are many triggers that can provoke or aggravate a migraine attack. Tiredness, stress, depression, shock, loud noises, bright lights and diet have all been implicated.

It is not only the types of foods we eat in our diet that are important, but also the frequency of our meals. Long gaps between meals can trigger a migraine due to the lowering of the blood sugar level. It is therefore important to have regular meals and snacks, particularly before strenuous exercise, such as bread, pasta, rice and potatoes, and proteins such as meat, fish, cheese, eggs and pulses. Sugary foods – for example, sweets and chocolates – provide only temporary relief, as they cause a rapid rise, followed by a rapid fall in blood sugar levels.

A study conducted in Chicago in 2003 in children and adolescents showed that diet can play an important role in causing headaches and migraine. The foods that most commonly triggered attacks were cheese, chocolate, hot-dogs, monosodium glutamate, aspartame, fatty foods, ice-cream, red wine and beer. These foods contain amines such as tyramine which, when they are absorbed into the body, may change the diameter of small blood vessels. This can bring on a migraine attack. The amines are absorbed more easily when fat is present. Other foods, such as citrus fruit and caffeine, were also implicated.

A study carried out by Professor Soothill at Great Ormond Street Children's Hospital in London showed a dramatic reduction in frequency of migraine attacks in children following an exclusion diet. He also found that these children had a problem with only a small number of foods.

Therefore, for migraine suffers we recommend that an exclusion diet should be tried (see page 31).

Asthma

Asthma is becoming increasingly common worldwide. The main symptoms are wheezing and difficulty in breathing, which may be accompanied by coughing. It is thought that many cases are caused by exposure to allergens in early life, especially dust mite, and pet allergens such as cat dander. Food intolerance may be particularly important in severe or brittle asthma, where as many as 65 per cent of patients have been found to have attacks after eating certain foods, the most important being wheat and dairy products. As asthma attacks may be very serious, asthmatics, particularly children, should embark on an exclusion diet only under medical supervision.

Eczema

Eczema, also known as atopic dermatitis, is an itching red rash often found on the inside of the elbow and knee. The rash tends to come and go, and may scale over and form a crust. It is often treated with steroid creams and antihistamine pills. Eczema is particularly common in young infants and children, who frequently also suffer from asthma or rhinitis.

Studies have indicated that eczema can be caused by food intolerance, possibly of an allergic nature. In children, the more severe the eczema, the more likely it is that food hypersensitivity is playing a role. Approximately a third of children with mild to moderate eczema are found to have food hypersensitivity. The most common foods involved are eggs and milk, but peanuts, soya, wheat and fish may also contribute to symptoms. In children with severe eczema 60 per cent are found to react to one or more of these foods. However, 85 per cent of young infants with eczema outgrow their food sensitivity by their third birthday. With your doctor's agreement a milk- and egg-free diet may be a sensible first approach. This must be closely supervised by a state-registered dietitian.

In adults, food sensitivity appears to be less common, with other factors such as house-dust mites, pollen, animal fur and moulds playing a more important role.

Urticaria

Urticaria (or nettle rash) is a common condition in which large itchy red blotches appear anywhere on the skin. In some cases sufferers may also develop angioedema – painless and sometimes itchy swelling, particularly of the lips and mouth. Very occasionally, this can be life-threatening, if the throat becomes inflamed. These symptoms can last for as little as one to two hours or they may persist for many months, known as chronic urticaria.

Urticaria can occur at any age and in both sexes, but chronic urticaria is more common in adult women. The condition is usually treated with antihistamines. A number of factors can bring on urticaria, such as heat, pressure, water, cold, sunlight and physical exercise. However, in some cases foods are known to provoke an attack, the most common being cow's milk, fish, eggs, cheese, yeast, chocolate and caffeine. Artificial preservatives and colourings were thought to be important in causing urticaria but studies in 2003 and 2004 indicated that these were responsible in only 1–2 per cent of cases.

However, we recommend that those suffering from urticaria should begin by trying a diet free from artificial colourings, preservatives and salicylates (see Appendix B).

If there is no improvement in the condition after one month, an exclusion diet should be tried (see page 31).

Rhinitis

Rhinitis is a non-infectious disorder in which the sufferer has a persistently runny and stuffy nose. Like asthma, rhinitis has sometimes been found to be related to food. In one study of patients with rhinitis, two-thirds were shown to be affected by food. In 19 per cent of these cases, food was found to be the sole cause of the rhinitis. In some patients the rhinitis was caused by various inhaled allergens, but with food also having an effect. Dairy products, and food additives such as sodium benzoate, are common dietary causes of rhinitis, and, if your doctor is in agreement, it is certainly worth trying an exclusion diet.

Cow's milk sensitive enteropathy

This mainly affects babies who are bottle-fed before the age of four months. The symptoms are severe stomach pain (known as colic), diarrhoea, eczema, vomiting and a runny nose. Babies usually grow out of these once they are on a solid diet, at about the age of two.

Mothers who think their children are reacting to cow's milk should talk to their family doctor. Although a cow's milk-free diet may be suggested by a doctor or paediatrician, children should never be put on any abnormal diet without close medical supervision.

Arthritis

Many people are confused about the meaning of the word arthritis. It means swelling of the joints and there are numerous forms of arthritis, which may be caused by diseases as different as damage to the nerves or bleeding into the joints. No diet can help all these conditions.

Osteoarthritis is probably the most common form of arthritis, especially among women. It is believed to be caused by wear and tear of the joints, particularly in the hips and knees. This sort of arthritis will not be helped by diet unless, of course, weight reduction has been recommended by your doctor, to alleviate the pressure on the joints.

Gout is caused by sharp crystals of uric acid forming in the joints. The uric acid comes from the breakdown of chemicals known as purines. Although most doctors now treat gout with drugs, which block the formation of uric acid or increase its excretion in the urine, some still supplement these with a diet which avoids foods rich in purines. These are found in protein-rich foods, in particular offal (e.g. liver, kidneys), peas, beans, sardines, pilchards, anchovies, herrings and fish roes. Gout was therefore one of the original forms of arthritis to be treated by diet. Treating rheumatoid arthritis by diet is not so simple.

Rheumatoid arthritis is a disease of the connective tissues, particularly affecting the tissues around the joints. It causes inflammation and, eventually, stiffening of the joint concerned. This form of arthritis is more common among women than men and affects up to 38 women per 1,000 of the population at some time in their lives.

This is the form of arthritis that has caused the most interest and controversy as far as diet is concerned. Several different diets have been promoted by doctors and herbalists but, unfortunately, none has proved to be entirely successful. Although a number of doctors have reported that a few of their patients with rheumatoid arthritis have definitely found that foods caused their problems, a large number seem to improve for a short time only. This may be because of a placebo effect – if they think the treatment is doing them good, then it will. In studies where diet has proved successful, patients have often reported that they suffered other food-related symptoms.

Psoriatic arthritis is a special type of arthritis that sometimes affects people with the skin disease psoriasis. The arthritis affects the lining of the joints, causing swelling, pain and stiffness. It usually affects only a few joints in the body. We have found considerable success in treating this.

We therefore suggest that if you have rheumatoid or psoriatic arthritis, a diet is well worth a try. We recommend the LOFFLEX diet, which is explained in detail in the chapter on Crohn's disease, but with the slight change that red meats, including beef, lamb and pork, should be excluded. If there is initial improvement, subsequent food reintroduction should proceed in the same way, as discussed on page 63. It is very important for anyone following the diet not to stop taking any pills that have been prescribed until it is quite clear that the diet has relieved the symptoms. If you stop taking medication too early you may suffer considerable pain. Again, we emphasise that it is essential to obtain your doctor's agreement before starting a trial to discover whether your arthritis can be helped by diet.

Food supplements for arthritis

There are many supplements recommended for arthritis sufferers. The two most common supplements are fish oils and evening primrose oil.

The fatty acids found in oily fish such as mackerel, herrings, sardines, salmon and trout are used by the body to make chemicals which are less inflammatory than those made from fats in a normal diet. In this way the fish oil has a mild anti-inflammatory effect which may make it possible for people to take fewer drugs. Cod liver oil has been taken by arthritis sufferers for years; many people mistakenly believing that it 'oils their joints' and, thus, makes them more mobile. Scientific studies have shown some benefit for people suffering from rheumatoid arthritis when used in a concentrated form. Unfortunately, cod liver oil capsules from a pharmacist may not be concentrated enough to produce the same benefits.

Also, the supplements used must be taken over a long period of time, at least three to six months, to be effective. However, if you are taking a cod liver oil supplement, *do not* exceed the manufacturer's dose as you could actually do yourself more harm than good.

Evening primrose oil acts in a very similar way to fish oil to produce an anti-inflammatory effect. However, there seems to be no advantage in taking both oils at the same time.

Other supplements often recommended for arthritis include ginseng, royal jelly, cider vinegar, New Zealand green-lipped mussel extract, selenium, garlic, honey and various vitamin supplements. These have not been scientifically studied and it is difficult to say whether they have any benefit. Often they are expensive to buy and may have harmful side-effects if taken in larger doses for a long period of time.

Arthritis: testing by diet

As we mentioned earlier, many different diets have been claimed to relieve rheumatoid arthritis. They are often based on diets eaten in countries where arthritis is rare. Unfortunately, most of these have been found to be disappointing.

Dr Dong's diet was devised in the 1940s and is based on a typical diet from China, where arthritis is relatively unusual. It is rich in fish and excludes red meat, fruits, egg yolk, dairy produce, additives, spices and chocolate. Although many people have claimed that the diet has helped them, a controlled trial failed to reveal any differences between those who followed Dong and those who ate an ordinary diet.

We believe that this diet excludes too many foods to be followed happily for a long time, and it lacks the flexibility of the exclusion diet – there is no point in avoiding a food unless you are quite sure that eating it causes trouble.

Because Eskimos eat a lot of fish, and very few of them suffer from arthritis, it has been suggested that enriching the diet with the polyunsaturated fatty acids found in fish might help arthritis sufferers. However, a study reported in *The Lancet* showed that the benefit was limited. The treatment group had less morning stiffness and fewer tender joints after twelve weeks on this diet, but when they stopped it they appeared to deteriorate more quickly than the other group, who received the average American diet. Besides, the relief experienced during the diet was far from complete. In our view there is little point in following a restrictive diet if it does not give total benefit.

The acid-reducing diet is based on the idea that acids produced in the body during digestion cause arthritis. It is true that uric acid is formed in gout (see page 11) but there is little other evidence to back this theory. The acid-reducing diet differs from Dr Dong's in that it encourages dairy products and avoids fish, tea and coffee. Apart from this it is very similar and lacks scientific support.

Crohn's disease

The role of food intolerance and the dietary treatment of Crohn's disease is discussed in detail on page 57.

Hyperactivity

Many children behave badly and it has become almost fashionable to call a child hyperactive who is simply energetic and noisy. But there is a clear distinction between overactivity, which is due to excessive energy, and hyperactivity, a condition that needs special treatment.

Very few children suffer from hyperactivity. The majority who have the condition are boys aged between one and seven. They demonstrate a sustained increase in physical activity together with poor concentration, impulsive behaviour and temper tantrums. Associated with this condition may be poor eating and sleeping habits, abnormal thirst and learning and behavioural problems. Many also suffer from headaches, asthma, hay fever and catarrh.

The most famous findings about diet and hyperactivity were made by Dr Ben Feingold in the United States. His diet, based on the elimination of artificial colours and flavours, aspirin and natural salicylates found in some fruits and vegetables, helped 30 to 50 per cent of the children he was treating to improve. Hyperactivity is also linked to other factors such as chemicals (found in aerosols, disinfectants, perfume, etc.) and dust.

Many paediatricians working with hyperactive children have dismissed the Feingold diet and at present there seem to be as many arguments against treatment by diet as there are for it. However, a study at the Hospital for Sick Children in Great Ormond Street, London, reported success with dietary treatment carried out in children with this problem. Of the 76 children treated, 21 recovered, 41 improved and only 14 showed no improvement. These children were put on a much stricter diet than Dr Feingold's. Not only additives, but foods such as cow's milk, chocolate, wheat, oranges, cheese and eggs were shown to affect the children. Sugar, which had been blamed by many previous researchers, was found to affect very few of the children.

With a child known to be hyperactive it would seem reasonable to start on the exclusion diet (see page 31). This excludes all the relevant foods and, by reintroducing the foods as instructed, the solution may be found. When dealing with growing children it is, of course, especially important to make sure that sufficient food, minerals and vitamins are provided. For example, calcium supplements may be necessary if a suitable milk substitute is not used.

Some parents may wish to try a diet based on Dr Feingold's original observations, and we include an artificial colouring-, preservative- and salicylate-free diet in Appendix B.

Please note that a child should undertake an exclusion diet only with the approval, and under the supervision, of a medical specialist. The final diet must always be checked by a trained dietitian.

Autism

Children with autism spectrum disorder (ASD) frequently complain of gastrointestinal symptoms that may resolve with an exclusion diet, together with apparent improvement of some of the behavioural symptoms. Researchers in Minnesota have discovered that some children with ASD have immune reactions to dietary proteins that are partly associated with abnormal immune responses to toxins produced by gut bacteria. Elimination of milk and wheat from the diet has been shown to help these children and such a diet may reduce abnormal chemicals excreted in the urine at the same time as behaviour and social skills improve. However, other foods as well as food additives may also be involved and, in the first instance, we suggest a trial of the exclusion diet.

Please note that a child should undertake an exclusion diet only with the approval, and under the supervision, of a medical specialist. The final diets must always be checked by a state-registered dietitian.

Testing for food intolerance

The main difficulty in treating patients with food intolerance is that the foods concerned vary greatly from one patient to another. Nearly all patients with coeliac disease will improve on a gluten-free diet; however, some patients with IBS may be better if they avoid chocolate and peanuts, whereas others are affected by dairy products. This variation causes much confusion. In order to simplify the problem, doctors have tried to find a reliable method of testing for food intolerance. We describe some of these techniques below; so far, all have proved disappointing.

Skin tests were developed by the classical allergists of the early twentieth century. An extract of a suspected food is injected into the skin, either by putting a small quantity on the skin and pricking through, or by injecting a small amount immediately beneath the skin (this is called an intradermal injection). If the test is positive, the site of the injection will swell up and be surrounded by an area of inflammation. As only one skin prick is necessary for each food, a whole battery of tests may be done at the same sitting.

This type of test may be very useful when someone suffers from a genuine food allergy, but it will not cause a reaction in anyone who is, for example, lacking the enzyme that breaks down milk sugar. Despite a negative skin test, such a person would still show symptoms after drinking milk. Many people with food-related conditions such as migraine, diarrhoea and hyperactivity may have a negative skin test result.

As most people don't know the mechanisms by which their food is upsetting them, and as skin tests of this sort are by and large only available in private clinics, which are expensive, they are probably not the best tests to begin with.

The tongue test is a modification of the skin test. Here the food extract is placed under the tongue to see if it provokes a reaction. We have found it to be disappointing and unreliable.

The radioallergosorbent test (RAST) is a more sophisticated form of the skin test. Blood from people with genuine food allergy contains antibodies to the foods concerned and these can be detected in the laboratory through a complex analysis. Again, this test will be negative for people who do not have a true allergy but who do have a food intolerance caused by a different mechanism. It has the same limited use as skin tests.

The cytotoxic test. In this test a sample of blood from the donor is mixed with food extracts. A few minutes later changes in the blood cells are observed under a microscope. As only a small quantity of blood and a small quantity of food extract are needed, a whole series of tests may be done on a single specimen of blood, so that the donor may be given a detailed report on possible food intolerances.

In theory, this test is enormously attractive, but we have found that in practice it, too, is of little help to people with intolerances. Researchers have not yet confirmed that the blood cells of people with food intolerance react against food chemicals, although they may in people who have true allergies. Most independent scientific studies have shown this test to be unreliable, and we have certainly found this to be the case. Many people come to see us claiming that they are unable to eat foods because their blood cells have reacted to samples of the foods in a cytotoxic test, but when they actually eat them, nothing untoward happens. For example, we gave wheat to a patient who agreed to do a 'blind' test. Although she had been told that she had a wheat intolerance, she had no reaction at all when she was given wheat to eat without knowing.

The hair test. Many laboratories offer to diagnose your food intolerances by analysing the minerals in a specimen of your hair. Minerals such as mercury, cadmium and arsenic are deposited in your hair as it grows. It is thought that a deficiency of a mineral can explain why some people react to certain foods. The amount of minerals in your hair sometimes reflects the amount in your body at the time the hair was formed – but of course in the case of people with long hair, this may have been many months before.

The link between mineral changes and food intolerances remains to be proved, and even if you have a hair analysis done you will still have to confirm yourself that the suspected foods cause trouble when you actually eat them. We do not recommend this technique. The main application of mineral analysis on hair is to detect the arsenic levels in murder victims!

Blood mineral analysis. A number of minerals are detectable in the blood and mineral analysis is offered by a number of laboratories on the same principle as detecting minerals in the hair. In practice, the significance of the levels of the various chemicals is poorly understood. Zinc is known to be very important for forming various enzymes and chemicals, and yet the way it works is still largely a mystery to us. Certainly, many people who are shown to have low levels of zinc in their blood in these tests don't appear to benefit when extra zinc is provided in their diet.

Since many of the other minerals being investigated are understood even less well than zinc, we do not have much faith in this type of mineral analysis for detecting food intolerance.

Food antibodies in the blood. As explained above, there are specific antibodies in the blood that allow the detection of genuine food allergies by the RAST test. This group of antibodies, which immunologists call IgE, is not present in food intolerances of other types. There is another group of antibodies called IgG, and in 2004 a research paper was published suggesting that these antibodies were valuable in identifying the foods responsible for intolerances. Patients' blood was tested and the levels of IgG food antibodies measured. The patients were then asked to follow diets avoiding the foods to which they had positive antibody tests. It was found that these patients improved significantly more than others who followed a 'sham' diet, in which they avoided foods against which no antibodies had been discovered. It was suggested that a simple blood test was thus all that was needed for patients to know which foods they should avoid.

In our opinion, however, IgG antibodies are not an accurate guide to food intolerances. As explained before, we have strong evidence that intolerances are often caused by bacteria in the gut, rather than by antibodies. What is more, IgG food antibodies may be found in the blood of healthy people who can eat any food without ill effects. We have suggested that the reason that the group of patients improved following diets based on antibody results was that many of them avoided wheat, whereas patients on the 'sham' diets did not. As can be seen from the table on page 29, wheat is by far the food most likely to upset patients, and is the likely reason for the differences between the two groups.

We believe that the only reliable way to detect food intolerances is to follow a carefully chosen but restricted diet, and see if symptoms improve. If they do, subsequent food reintroductions will show clearly which items can cause a recurrence of the original problem.

Irritable Bowel Syndrome and the Exclusion Diet

Some considerations before changing your diet

If your doctor has diagnosed irritable bowel syndrome, changing your diet may be the answer to your problems. However, before embarking on an exclusion diet it is worth considering simple changes to your diet and lifestyle that may have important implications on your well-being. For example:

Do you tend to skip meals and grab a snack when time permits?
Do you eat very quickly?
Are you drinking enough fluids?
Do you drink coffee or tea continually throughout the day?

It is important to treat your gut with respect. Developing a regular meal pattern will help your gut to establish its own routine. If meals are missed, the signals that regulate bowel movements become confused. A large meal on a stomach that has been starved most of the day may result in an exaggerated stimulus to the bowels, which in turn can lead to discomfort and diarrhoea. Try to spread your food intake more evenly throughout the day. If your stomach starts to feel uncomfortable, stop eating; save a dessert until later.

Some people find four or five smaller meals and snacks easier to manage than two or three large ones.

Take your time when you eat. Eating very quickly and drinking fluids at the same time makes it more likely that you will swallow a lot of air, leading to bloating and flatulence. Rushing around after eating diverts the blood away from your gut, which may disrupt digestion.

Try to have regular drinks, aiming for a minimum of eight cups or glasses a day. This is especially important if you suffer from constipation. Fibrous matter in the intestine absorbs water, making it swell. This produces a bulky stool, which helps stimulate the bowel to push contents through the system. If you are dehydrated, stools will be small and hard, making them difficult to expel. Try to include drinks such as water, fruit juice and squashes. Some people find that carbonated drinks cause distention and discomfort. Caffeine, found in coffee, tea and cola drinks, can act as a powerful stimulus to the gut and make it difficult to relax intestinal muscles. It also has a diuretic action, which has a dehydrating effect on the body. Try cutting down your caffeine intake and replacing such beverages with decaffeinated alternatives or herbal and fruit teas.

Certain foods can irritate the stomach. These may include very spicy foods, acidic foods such as citrus fruit and vinegar, or raw vegetables such as cucumber, peppers and onion. Alcohol may act as an irritant, especially on an empty stomach. Fried or very rich foods are also common causes of indigestion and heartburn. Another important point to consider is whether you are eating too little or too much fibre and this is discussed in more detail a little later.

Be aware that there may be factors other than food that are having an effect on your digestive system. The most important of these is probably stress. The connection between mind and gut is very strong and during stressful periods the intestine may be over-stimulated, making it difficult to function normally. Are your symptoms worse during the week, improving at the weekend or when you go on holiday? This may suggest a link with stress or it may reflect differences in eating patterns or types of food eaten.

It is not uncommon for people to hyperventilate without being aware that they are doing so. During the day large volumes of air can be swallowed in this way, resulting in bloating and discomfort. A physiotherapist can advise you on exercises to help you to breathe normally again.

Some women find their pattern of symptoms is related to their menstrual cycle and thus changes in hormone levels are likely to be playing a significant role.

It may help to keep a diary of when and what you eat and drink alongside a record of your symptoms. Include details such as periods of increased stress and the stage of your menstrual cycle. This should help you determine whether there are any links between these factors and your symptoms.

Fibre – too much or not enough?

High-fibre diets

A high-fibre diet includes wholegrain breads and cereals, vegetables, pulses (beans, lentils and peas), fruit, nuts and seeds. Foods containing fibre are important contributors of vitamins and minerals that make up a balanced diet. In addition, fibre itself has an important role. As explained earlier, it acts by absorbing fluids from the gut which causes it to swell. This produces a soft, easily passed stool. Increased stool bulk also helps stimulate the bowel wall to contract and push the contents through.

Not surprisingly, constipation-predominant IBS is the most likely variant to respond to an increase in fibre. The Western diet has a tendency to be low in fibre, owing to easily available highly processed and convenience foods. Dietary fibre should be increased gradually by including one or two new high-fibre foods each week. Rather than simply adding bran to foods, try adding a variety of fruit, vegetable and cereal sources. This ensures a good mixture of soluble fibre (found in certain fruits and vegetables, pulses and oats) and insoluble fibre (found mainly in cereal products), each of which has different beneficial effects on bowel function. It is important that you increase fluid intake at the same time as increasing fibre.

A high-fibre diet tends to be the first-line treatment recommended for IBS. There is, however, no evidence to suggest that people with IBS consume less fibre than those without. Fibre does not necessarily help all symptoms of IBS. In fact, some people find that their IBS becomes worse when they eat a high-fibre diet, especially when the fibre is in the form of bran. This is because fibre can act as an irritant. It is fermented in the large bowel by bacteria, which produce gas. If too much gas is produced, it can lead to bloating, flatulence and discomfort. Too much fibre may also aggravate diarrhoea, as it speeds up the passage of food through the gut. A high-fibre diet should be tried for about four weeks to see if it is helpful. If the constipation is not resolved or if the high-fibre diet is not well tolerated, alternative types of fibre may be useful. These are known as bulking agents and are discussed on page 25.

Low-fibre diets

If you suffer from diarrhoea, bloating and flatulence, you may find a reduction in dietary fibre helpful. A low-fibre diet (outlined on page 25) works by reducing fermentation in the large bowel.

The low-fibre diet should be followed for four weeks. If you do not notice an improvement in your symptoms or you feel worse after this time, you should return to your normal diet. If, however, you are feeling better, you should try to reintroduce some fibre back into your diet following the guidelines on page 26. You may find that you tolerate some types of fibre better than others and you will therefore need to reintroduce these separately to note the effect. Build up the fibre to a level that you can tolerate. If you are unable to reintroduce much fibre you may need a vitamin and mineral supplement to ensure your diet is balanced, and this should be discussed with a dietitian.

Bulking agents

It may be necessary to take a bulking agent while on a low-fibre diet to prevent constipation from developing. This should be discussed with your doctor. Bulking agents are natural sources of fibre that cannot be broken down to any great extent by bacteria in the gut. This means that they have the useful property of encouraging regular bowel movements but – in contrast to cereal, vegetable and fruit fibre – do not contribute to the production of gas. There are several suitable varieties including Celevac (methylcellulose), Normacol (sterculia) or cracked linseed, which is available from health food shops. We no longer recommend laxatives based on isphagula husk (Fybogel, Regulan, psyllium) as this is sometimes a cause of gas and bloating. If one variety does not appear to help it is worth trying an alternative. It is essential that extra fluids are taken with these preparations.

The low-fibre diet

Eat your normal amount of meat, fish, eggs, milk and dairy products, fats and oils. These do not contain any fibre. For cereal products, fruits and vegetables, follow the guidelines below.

	Not allowed	*Allowed*
Cereal	Wholemeal, granary and brown bread, bran, wholemeal flour and foods made with these	White bread, white flour and foods made with these

	Not allowed	Allowed
	Wholemeal pasta, brown rice	White pasta, white rice
	Wholegrain breakfast cereals, e.g. Weetabix, All-Bran, porridge, muesli and any cereals with added nuts and dried fruit	Rice Krispies and Cornflakes
	Wholegrain biscuits, e.g. digestive, flapjacks and cereal bars; biscuits containing nuts and dried fruit	Biscuits made from white flour, e.g. Rich Tea, wafers
	Wholegrain crackers and crispbreads, Ryvita, oatcakes	Crispbreads and crackers made from white flour, e.g. cream crackers
Fruit	All dried fruit, berries and bananas	All other fruit, maximum 2 portions a day; avoid skins and seeds
Vegetables	All pulses, beans, chickpeas, lentils, peas, sweetcorn, Brussels sprouts	All other vegetables, maximum 2 portions a day in addition to potato; avoid skins, seeds and stalks
Miscellaneous	Nuts, seeds	Fruit and vegetable juices (not prune juice)

Reintroducing fibre

Week 1

Try eating the skins on fruit and vegetables, e.g. apples, pears, potatoes.

Week 2

Eat an extra piece of fruit a day, e.g. a banana (but not

dried fruit), *or* an extra portion of vegetables (not pulses). Five portions a day of fruits and vegetables (not including potatoes) are recommended long-term for a healthy diet. N.B. One glass of fruit juice counts as one portion of fruit.

Week 3
Try replacing white bread with wholemeal bread.

Week 4
Try a higher-fibre breakfast cereal, e.g. Weetabix, Shredded Wheat or Bran Flakes.

Week 5
If you are still symptom-free, you may like to try dried fruit or pulses.

Remember, these reintroductions give a gradual build-up of fibre in your diet. The aim is to identify a level of fibre that you can comfortably take.
You may find that you can eat high-fibre vegetables on days when you do not have wholemeal bread and high-fibre breakfast cereals, or vice versa. If this is the case, try varying the sources of your fibre intake on a daily basis to achieve a balanced diet.

The exclusion diet – an introduction

If you have found previous suggestions unhelpful, now might be the time to consider whether a specific food or group of foods make your symptoms worse. An exclusion diet will help you find out whether you have any food intolerances. It can be difficult to pinpoint individual foods because the ones that are most likely to upset you are the ones that we tend to eat every day, sometimes at every meal. If your symptoms are similar from day to day this will provide few clues as to the offending foods. Also, a food may need to be eaten more than once before symptoms are experienced and reactions may not develop for several hours or even until the following day.

Although some foods are more likely to be responsible for food-related symptoms than others, the only way to decide which foods upset you is to test them individually. Excluding one food at a time may not be helpful if you have more than one food intolerance. For this reason a safe, simple diet containing none of the common problem foods needs to be followed for a two-week period. If at the end of this you feel there has been a definite improvement in your symptoms, reintroduce the foods one at a time. If, however, you feel there has been little or no change, you should stop the diet and return to your normal diet. The next section will guide you through the exclusion and reintroduction stages of the diet.

How the diet was developed

Altogether, 584 patients with IBS took part in studies we carried out to develop the exclusion diet. Between 1979 and 1982 we studied 182 patients, using a very restrictive few-foods diet followed by the gradual reintroduction and testing of foods. One hundred and twenty-two patients reported a relief of their symptoms on this diet. A list was drawn up of the foods that upset these patients (see page 29). From this list we developed a less restrictive exclusion diet that avoided all the foods to which 20 per cent or more of the patients had been intolerant. This list was modified slightly following two subsequent reviews of the diet to produce the diet we now recommend. Approximately 60 per cent of all the patients who took part in the studies and completed food testing found they were able to control their symptoms on this diet.

Review of foods tested by patients attending clinic, 1979–1982

Food	Percentage of patients affected	Food	Percentage of patients affected
Cereals		**Vegetables**	
wheat	60	onions	22
corn	44	potatoes	20
oats	34	cabbage	19
rye	30	sprouts	18
barley	24	peas	17
rice	15	carrots	15
		lettuce	15
Dairy Products		leeks	15
milk	44	broccoli	14
cheese	39	soya beans	13
eggs	26	spinach	13
butter	25	mushrooms	12
yoghurt	24	parsnips	12
		tomatoes	11
Fish		cauliflower	11
white fish	10	celery	11
shellfish	10	green beans	10
smoked fish	7	cucumber	10
		turnip/swede	10
Meat		marrow	8
beef	16	beetroot	8
pork	14	peppers	6
chicken	13		
lamb	11	**Miscellaneous**	
turkey	8	coffee	33
		tea	25
Fruit		nuts	22
citrus	24	chocolate	22
rhubarb	12	preservatives	20
apple	12	yeast	20
banana	11	sugar cane	13
pineapple	8	sugar beet	12
pear	8	alcohol	12
strawberries	8	saccharin	9
grapes	7	honey	2
melon	5		
avocado	5		
raspberries	4		

Getting started

Before starting the exclusion diet, discuss your symptoms with your doctor to make sure he or she thinks this approach is sensible. Check that your doctor agrees that you have one of the conditions that can be helped by diet: it may be that you have another problem, which has similar symptoms but needs different treatment. You should also discuss with your doctor whether or not you should continue with any pills or medicines that you have been taking. In general it is better to take as few pills as possible while trying an exclusion diet, as many contain starches as fillers, and they may be part of the problem.

First, consider how long it will take you to complete the diet and when would be the best time to start. The basic diet takes just two weeks but if you improve you will need to begin the gradual reintroduction of foods into your diet. This may take two to three months, depending on how many foods cause problems. It may, for example, be better to delay starting until a holiday or a particularly busy social period is out of the way. Be prepared to make some sacrifices; in the early stages of the diet take-aways are generally not recommended and it can be very difficult to eat out at restaurants.

You will also need to think about how you can fit an exclusion diet around work. It is unlikely that staff canteens or sandwich shops will provide suitable meals and you will therefore have to take your own food to work. You may also need to allow a little more time for lunch instead of having a quick snack on the run.

Balancing the exclusion diet with family life is another consideration. Will your family eat the same meals as you or will it involve cooking separate meals? Following a diet can be time-consuming: you will have to plan each meal, and cooking is likely to take longer, because few convenience foods are suitable. However, the recipes at the back of this book have been designed to make cooking on the exclusion diet as quick and easy as possible.

If you are vegetarian you may need to spend a little more time planning what you are going to eat as several of the staple foods of a vegetarian diet, such as dairy products, eggs and nuts, are excluded. Eat a wide variety of the vegetarian foods that are allowed to ensure your diet remains balanced, including a good mixture of protein sources from soya products, pulses, cereals and seeds.

On the positive side, following the exclusion diet is the best way to find out whether food is at the root of your problems. If it is successful, you will have found a cure to your symptoms that does not involve any medication. You will also have an opportunity to take a fresh look at your diet and to experiment with new tastes. You may even find you lose a few pounds in weight in the process!

The exclusion diet

For the first two weeks of the exclusion diet, you should avoid all the foods in the 'Not allowed' column and replace them with those in the 'Allowed' column.

	Not allowed	Allowed
Meat	Beef, meat products, e.g. sausages, beefburgers, meat pies, pâtés	All other meat and poultry, e.g. chicken, turkey, lamb, pork (including ham and bacon), liver, kidney
Fish	Fish in batter, crumb or tinned in vegetable oil	All other fresh, smoked and tinned fish, shellfish
Vegetables	Potatoes, onion, sweetcorn, baked beans	Sweet potatoes, all other vegetables, including salad and pulses
Fruit	Citrus fruit, e.g. oranges, lemons, grapefruit	All other fruit, fresh, tinned and dried

	Not allowed	*Allowed*
Cereals	Wheat, oats, rye, corn, barley (see pages 262–265 for foods containing these)	Rice, rice cakes, ground rice, Rice Krispies, rice noodles, rice pasta, tapioca, sago, arrowroot
Cooking oils	Corn oil, vegetable oil (may contain corn oil), nut oils	Sunflower, soya, olive, rapeseed, safflower oils
Dairy products	Cow's, goat's and sheep's milk and products, butter, margarine, cream, cheese, yoghurt, ice-cream, eggs (see pages 261–262 for foods containing these)	Soya milk and products e.g. dairy-free margarine, tofu, soya yoghurt, soya cream and soya ice-cream, sorbet (non-citrus); check labels
Beverages	Tea, coffee (including decaffeinated), squashes and fizzy drinks, citrus fruit juice, alcohol, tap water	Herbal and fruit teas, Ribena, non-citrus fruit juices, e.g. apple, pineapple, tomato, mineral water
Miscellaneous	Yeast (see page 264 for foods containing this) salad cream and dressings, mustard, vinegar, tinned or packet sauces, chocolate, sweets, nuts	Salt, pepper, herbs, spices in moderation (see page 49 and recipe section for alternative gravies, sauces and dressings); sugar, honey, syrup, jam (non-citrus), carob, Kendal mint cake, seeds, (e.g. Sesame snaps, halva, tahini).

Following an exclusion diet

Here are a few points to help guide you through the diet:

1. For two weeks before starting, record all the symptoms you have had, and when, to help judge the value of the diet later on.
2. For the first two weeks of the exclusion diet keep strictly to the list of allowed foods on pages 31–32. Remember, it is essential to continue for two weeks; because all traces of offending foods eaten before the diet begins must disappear from the body before symptoms clear, improvement is rarely seen in the first week. Don't give up; if you take a day off you will have wasted all your previous efforts, and will have to start again from the beginning.
3. During the first fortnight it is wise to exclude any foods besides those listed on pages 31–32 that you suspect have upset you; later on you will test and assess them properly.
4. During the second week you should eat as wide a variety of the 'allowed' foods as possible. This will help you notice any unusual food intolerances.
5. Throughout the two weeks keep an accurate diary of everything you eat and drink, which symptoms you have and when. Use a small notebook and allow a spread of two pages for each day (see below).
6. If after two weeks your symptoms have not improved, it is unlikely that food intolerance is the cause of your problems. Go back to normal eating, and ask your doctor about trying a different treatment.
7. If your symptoms have resolved you should proceed to the next stage of the diet: food reintroduction (page 34). If your symptoms have partially improved it may be helpful to continue the diet for just one further week, using your food and symptoms diary to help identify any further food intolerances. Start to test foods only if you feel there has been an obvious change in your symptoms; otherwise, return to your normal diet.

Example of a food and symptom diary

	Foods	Symptoms
Breakfast 8.00 am	Rice Krispies, soya milk, apple juice	8.30 am Diarrhoea
Mid-morning 11.00am	Banana, peppermint tea	12.15 pm Wind
Lunch 1.15 pm	Chicken drumsticks, rice salad, lettuce, tomato, cucumber, soya yoghurt	2.30 pm Headache started
Mid-afternoon 4.00 pm	Camomile tea, pear	
Supper 7.30 pm	Pork chops, sweet potatoes, peas, carrots, soya rice pudding, Ribena	8.45 pm Bloated stomach 9.15 pm Diarrhoea

Reintroducing foods

Hopefully, by now you are feeling delighted by the improvement that the diet has brought. It is now highly likely that your symptoms can be controlled by diet. However, to find out exactly which foods are responsible still requires very careful planning. Continue to keep your diary throughout the reintroduction phase. The list on pages 36–37 shows the order for reintroduction. Try to keep to the following rules for reintroducing foods:

• With irritable bowel syndrome, migraine, asthma and rhinitis, we recommend that you reintroduce one food every two days. For constipation-predominant irritable bowel syndrome it may be wise to extend this period to four days.

In the cases of eczema and urticaria a longer period of a week is recommended.

- Eat plenty of the foods that you are testing. Have at least two good helpings a day or the quantity specified in the reintroduction list. If after the last test day there are no ill-effects you may assume that the food is safe to eat and therefore you can include it as normal in your diet.
- If you have a reaction stop eating the food you are testing immediately. The time it takes to recover from a reaction varies. Do not test any new foods until you are completely well again; otherwise it will be difficult to tell if any symptoms experienced are due to the new food or left over from the previous food. Do not try to rush through the list of foods – the more haste, the less speed. The average reintroduction time is two months; it will be longer if you react to several foods.
- The time it takes for symptoms to show also varies. Do not expect symptoms to develop immediately after eating a food. It may take 24 to 48 hours for a reaction to show. Sometimes symptoms appear so slowly that they are hardly noticeable to begin with. This is why it is important to keep a diary – you can look back and see when you were last really well and this will help you spot the offending food.
- Drink plenty of water to help recover from a reaction. Some people find that adding a little bicarbonate of soda increases the effectiveness of this treatment. If you need any painkillers, take only the soluble preparations of paracetamol or Solpadeine.
- Some foods are made up of more than one ingredient. These ingredients will need to be tested separately as, if a reaction occurs, you will not know which ingredient caused it. For example, bread is made from yeast and wheat. You will need to test yeast first before you can test the wheat in bread.
- Try to introduce foods in the order that they appear in the list on pages 36–37. You may miss out a food that you never eat, but if it is included as an ingredient of another food that you eat you should still test it. For example, you

may not eat a boiled or fried egg, but you may consume an egg as a cake ingredient. Foods eaten only occasionally can be moved to the end of the list, but do not forget to test them. If you suspect a food upsets you, you should still test it in case you have identified it wrongly.

- Take a week to test wheat, as symptoms often develop slowly and may be missed. For the first four days test white wheat products such as white flour, white pasta and white bread (if yeast is tolerated). For the remaining three days try testing higher-fibre wheat products including wholemeal or granary bread and breakfast cereals such as Weetabix or Shreddies. It is wise to leave the testing of wheat until late in the reintroductions, when you have a little experience under your belt.

- Sometimes you may suspect that a food upsets you, but are not absolutely sure. Don't waste time testing and retesting one food; leave it out for a few weeks and come back to it later, when your diet is less restricted.

- At the end of the reintroductions you must go back and retest all foods you believe affect you. Some suspected reactions may have been coincidental and there is no point in avoiding a food unless you really have to.

Order of food reintroduction

Test each food for two days. Test at least twice per day or as indicated below.

Tap water	– take throughout the day
Potatoes	– e.g. baked, boiled, mashed (without dairy products)
Milk	– 450 ml throughout the day
Yeast	– take three Brewers' Yeast tablets (one with each meal) or two teaspoons fresh yeast spread on the rice cakes, each day
Tea	– take at least twice per day

Rye	– test Ryvita or rye bread (check bread is wheat-free), only test rye bread if yeast was tolerated
Beef	– e.g. have cold slices at lunch and steak, roast or mince in the evening
Butter or margarine	– e.g. spread on rice cakes, add to potato
Onions	– test cooked and raw
Eggs	– test two per day
Oats	– test porridge, oatcakes, flapjacks
Coffee	– test coffee beans and instant coffee
Chocolate	– test plain chocolate or cocoa
Citrus fruits	– test oranges, grapefruit, satsumas, etc., or orange juice
Corn	– test Cornflakes, cornflour, sweetcorn
Cheese	– try 60g (2 oz) twice a day
White wine	– test two glasses. If yeast is not tolerated, test spirits
Yoghurt	– test two small cartons a day
Wheat	– test for seven days taking wheat at each meal (see note on page 36 on how to test wheat)
Nuts	– try different varieties, 60g (2 oz) twice a day
Barley	– test barley flakes, pearl barley
Vinegar	– e.g. test on chips or in salad dressing

Frequently asked questions

Will my diet be nutritionally balanced?
Hopefully, you will need to avoid only one or two foods and will find your diet reasonably straightforward. If you are avoiding a number of foods, or a few important ones such as milk or wheat, ask your doctor to refer you to a dietitian to check that your diet is nutritionally balanced and to get ideas on replacement foods.

Try to eat a wide range of your safe foods rather than restricting yourself to a few. Check that you are following the guidelines for a balanced diet, outlined on page 51. If you are milk- and dairy product-intolerant you may not be getting enough calcium in your diet. Choose a calcium-enriched soya milk and include non-dairy sources of calcium in your diet such as tofu (soya bean curd), soya cheese, tinned fish (with bones), seeds, nuts, dried fruit, pulses, green vegetables and white bread. You may require a calcium supplement such as calcium gluconate or calcium carbonate, available from chemists. Discuss this with your doctor or dietitian.

If you are avoiding a number of foods you may benefit from a multivitamin or a multivitamin and mineral supplement such as Centrum, Sanatogen Gold or Forceval. Again, discuss this with your doctor or dietitian and check that the supplement is free of any ingredients that upset you, such as wheat, yeast, corn or milk. It is inadvisable to take large doses of individual vitamins and minerals as these are wasted if they exceed the amount required by the body and may even be toxic.

Will I be able to eat the foods that upset me again?
A reliable way to rid people of their food intolerances has not yet been found. Several methods have been tried, such as administering small quantities of the food as drops under the tongue or as an injection into the skin (known as enzyme-potentiated desensitization). Various drugs have also been tried. However, these have all produced disappointing results. We are now investigating whether supplementing the diet with various types of healthy bacteria can correct the fermentation of foods in the bowel. This is still in experimental stages. For now, while the intolerance continues, you will have to resign yourself to excluding the upsetting foods – as long as that seems preferable to suffering the symptoms.

However, many people find that after avoiding a food for several months it no longer upsets them, so recheck your food intolerances periodically – every six months, say – and you may be pleasantly surprised.

Could I develop more food intolerances?
Intolerances can change; just as intolerances can disappear, occasionally new ones can develop. Operations, courses of antibiotics, virus infections and bouts of gastroenteritis are some of the reasons for this happening. It may be easy for you to identify a food that has brought back your symptoms but if not, you will need to take yourself through the basic two-week diet and testing again.

What should I do if I have many food intolerances?
If you are unlucky and find that a large number of foods upset you, you should think seriously about whether it's worth trying to control your symptoms by diet. You should certainly ask your doctor to refer you to a dietitian who can check the nutritional value of what you are eating, and you should discuss other ways of coping with your symptoms with your doctor. If it is agreed that you can safely continue controlling your symptoms by diet rather than with drugs, it may help if you rotate your diet. We have found that when people can eat only a few foods, they eat so much of them that they may later get into trouble with these foods as well. Rotating your diet means that you eat foods from each food group only every three or four days, so that you are not over-exposed to any.

Below is an example of a rotating diet; you will obviously have to adapt it according to your particular intolerances. Check the recipe section for ideas on how to make interesting and varied meals from the foods listed.

	Day 1	*Day 2*	*Day 3*
Carbohydrate	rice, potato	millet, sweet potato	sago, buckwheat
Protein	poultry, beef	lamb, pulses	pork, fish
Vegetable	carrots, broccoli	parsnip, green beans	salad, courgette
Fruit	melon, pear	apple, mango	banana, pineapple

Common problems

Hunger!

If you are feeling hungry on the exclusion diet, it is probably because you are not replacing the foods you normally eat with suitable alternatives. In particular, you may not be eating enough of the starchy carbohydrate foods. Bread and potatoes are the main sources of starch in the British diet and without these you may have difficulty in satisfying your appetite. It is very important that you substitute these with alternative starchy carbohydrates at each meal. For example, breakfast should include rice cereal, rice cakes or one of the suggestions in the breakfast recipe section. For lunch, try a rice or buckwheat pasta salad or check the recipe section on snack lunches for some other ideas. Sweet potatoes are a good alternative to potatoes for your evening meal. Other substitutes for potato are listed on page 43. It is helpful always to have a home-made cake or biscuit (see recipes in baking section) at hand to silence a hungry stomach.

Losing weight

It is fairly common to lose a few pounds while on the exclusion diet, and for some this is an added bonus! A few people find they lose a lot of weight over a short period of time, which is likely to be due to fluid loss. Fluid retention can be a symptom of food intolerance and once the food or foods responsible are removed from the diet, the extra fluid is lost rapidly.

However, if you do not wish to lose weight or if you are losing weight too quickly, you will need to make some adjustments to your diet. Make sure you are having at least three substantial meals each day and include snacks (see recipes in baking section) in between. Try to follow the meal guidelines given on page 51. Increase your portion sizes of the carbohydrate foods such as rice, rice noodles and sweet potatoes, and of the protein foods (meat, fish and pulses) at both lunch and your evening meal. Try not to fill up on fruit and vegetables, since these will supply few calories. Include puddings regularly. Add milk-free margarine to rice cakes and sweet potatoes and use suitable oils to stir-fry meat and vegetables.

Tiredness

You may feel tired during the first few days of the diet, especially if you are used to drinking large amounts of coffee and tea, as these are stimulants. It is advisable to take things easy at the start of the diet. If the tiredness continues, it may be because you are not eating enough. In particular, you may need to eat more of the carbohydrate foods, as discussed above, which help to sustain your energy levels. If you are following the meal guidelines given on page 51 your diet should be well balanced and you should not need to take any extra vitamins or minerals. However, if you wish, you may take a multivitamin to see if this helps improve your energy levels. You should check that this supplement is free of wheat, corn or potato starch, and also milk and yeast. If you still feel tired you should ask your doctor to check whether you are anaemic.

Headaches

These are also common during the first few days of the diet, particularly if you are used to drinking a lot of coffee or tea. Try to avoid taking any painkillers, but if necessary use a soluble preparation such as soluble paracetamol or Solpadeine. If headaches continue make sure that you are drinking enough fluids (aim for ten cups or glasses a day) and that you are eating regular meals and snacks with carbohydrate-rich foods.

Worsening symptoms

You should find that you steadily improve during the second week of the diet. If your symptoms become worse, it is possible that you are intolerant to one of the foods normally found to be safe. If the symptoms are continual, the offending food is likely to be one which you are including daily, such as soya products or rice. You should try a few days without the suspected food to see if there is an improvement. If you do not feel any better, reintroduce that food and continue for a few more days, avoiding a different food. Another consideration is whether you are eating more fruit, vegetables or pulses (peas, beans and lentils) than normal, as too much fibre may trigger symptoms. If your symptoms are intermittent you should check through your diary for foods eaten within the previous 24 hours. Compare the foods you recorded with the list of foods on page 29. Foods that upset 10 to 20 per cent of patients are the most likely to be the cause. If you have eaten one of these you should avoid it and include it in the list of foods to test at the end of the two weeks.

Constipation

If you are used to eating wholegrain breakfast cereals and wholemeal bread you may find your fibre intake is lower on the exclusion diet, resulting in constipation. You will need to replace this fibre with other sources of fibre such as fruit, vegetables, pulses and grains such as millet and buckwheat. Constipation may also be a result of a reduced fluid intake. Make sure you replace the cups of tea and coffee you used to drink with similar amounts of other drinks. If the constipation does not resolve you may need to consider taking a bulking agent (see page 25). You should discuss the problem with your doctor.

Bloating and wind

In contrast, an increase in bloating and wind suggests you are eating too much fruit and vegetables, perhaps because you are struggling to find enough foods on the diet to fill up on. Try to keep to a maximum of two portions of fruit and two portions of vegetables (in addition to sweet potato) a day. Avoid pulses, dried fruit and brassicas (broccoli, cauliflower, cabbage and Brussels sprouts). If you find you need to eat high-fibre foods to prevent constipation, you may benefit from taking a bulking agent (see page 25).

Eating out

Eating out in the early stages of an exclusion diet is virtually impossible, unless the chef is particularly helpful. Similarly, all take-aways should be avoided. If it is difficult to avoid going out for a meal, keep to plain meat or fish, vegetables and rice (or potato once this has been introduced). Avoid sauces and eat fruit as a starter and dessert. If you eat a food that is not on the safe diet be prepared for symptoms the following day. You may need to delay reintroducing any foods for a few days until the symptoms have disappeared.

Experimenting with new foods

If you discover that you have food intolerances you cannot expect your diet to be just the same as ever, any more than you would expect food to be the same abroad as it is at home. You will have to be willing to experiment a little and get used to new tastes and textures. There are many substitutes for all the common ingredients such as potato, wheat and milk.

Alternatives to potatoes

Good alternatives to potatoes are the starchy root vegetables listed below. Other root vegetables such as swede, parsnip and turnip have a lower starch content and, although a valuable part of the diet, especially if combined with grains (see below), will not be as filling.

Sweet potatoes, which are yellow, orange or red in colour, are excellent potato substitutes, because they are very starchy and can be boiled, mashed, baked or fried in the same way as potatoes. They can usually be found in supermarkets. If you are boiling them, add a little lemon juice to the water to prevent discolouring (provided your diet permits it). Sweet potatoes are very good mashed and flavoured with cinnamon or nutmeg.

Yams have a faint nutty flavour. Cook and serve as for sweet potato. Yam flour is high in starch and can be used in casseroles, soups and for baking.

Eddoes or **taros** are eaten in the Pacific Islands and in parts of Africa and Asia. They have similar nutritional properties to potato and yam.

Cassava and **plantain** are other, less easily available substitutes for potato. These are staple foods eaten in some parts of South America, Africa and Asia.

Alternatively, potatoes can be replaced with rice or rice pasta or any of the grains listed below (without an asterisk).

Alternative grains and flours

The gluten in flours used for baking is elastic and holds air. This is why a strong (high-gluten) wheat flour is ideal for bread-making. Flours made from grains that are suitable for people with wheat intolerance are less likely to rise and great patience is needed to master the skills of baking (we give advice in the recipe section on baking).

Commercial gluten-free flours usually contain either wheat or corn starch. Therefore, if you are intolerant to either of these cereals, these flours will be unsuitable. They also tend to be very expensive.

Most of the flours listed are obtainable from wholefood or health-food shops, or may be milled from the grains in a powerful domestic blender. These are cheapest if bought in bulk from wholefood retailers. Best results are usually obtained by combining flours with different properties, as described below. **Flours that are not suitable for the initial two weeks of the exclusion diet are marked with an asterisk.**

Amaranth is an ancient grain originating from Mexico. It is in fact a seed which is ground into flour. High in protein, calcium and iron, it is best combined with a high-starch flour such as tapioca or potato for baking. It has a nutty flavour. Puffed amaranth may be used as a breakfast cereal.

Unfortunately, amaranth is becoming increasingly difficult to obtain in the UK.

Arrowroot is a starchy root with the consistency of cornflour. It is almost pure starch, providing little besides carbohydrate, and is most useful as a thickening agent for gravies and sauces.

Buckwheat is confusingly named, as it is unrelated to wheat and therefore perfectly safe to eat for those with wheat intolerance. The grain can be bought either roasted or unroasted, the roasted being stronger in flavour. Put the buckwheat into four times its volume of cold salted water, bring to the boil and simmer until the buckwheat is soft (about fifteen minutes). Do not stir while cooking. The flour, which has a strong and distinctive flavour, has an egg-like binding capacity which makes it very good in batters. It contains some protein and is rich in B vitamins and fibre. Some buckwheat products, for example spaghetti, are sold ready-made. Read the labels with special care as some also contain wheat flour.

Carob flour is ground from the pod of the locust tree and has a strong chocolate taste. As well as being high in pectin, it contains appreciable amounts of protein, carbohydrate, calcium and phosphorus. It is an invaluable alternative to chocolate for flavouring cakes and drinks.

****Chestnut flour** is derived from the sweet chestnut. It has a distinctive flavour and is rather heavy, but can be used for baking cakes and biscuits (for example, shortbread, scones and fruit crumbles).

Gram flour is made from ground chickpeas and is therefore high in fibre. It is widely used in Indian breads and batters and is high in protein, vitamins and minerals. It has a strong flavour and will become bitter if kept too long.

****Maize** (or **cornflour**) is a good thickening agent. It may be used in cakes, biscuits and bread, or for the Italian dish, polenta.

Millet, like rice, is a member of the grass family, but both are distant enough relatives of wheat to be safe for many people with wheat intolerance. It has good nutritional value, providing B vitamins, minerals and protein. Millet is available as a grain, flake or flour. It can be used in a variety of sweet and savoury dishes. Cook as for buckwheat. In some savoury dishes millet can be dry roasted in the pan first to enhance the flavour.

*Potato flour,** sometimes called fecule or farina, is an excellent thickening agent and is useful for baking when mixed with other flours. It is a pure starch with little flavour of its own. (Instant mashed potato is not a pure potato flour and should not be used as a substitute.)

Quinoa is a seed which can be used as a substitute for rice in savoury or sweet dishes. It has a mild nutty flavour. Originating from South America, it is high in protein, E and B vitamins and fibre. Before cooking, rinse thoroughly in cold water. Then cook as for rice for about ten minutes or according to instructions.

Rice flour, rice flakes and ground rice can be used for baking cakes and making puddings. Rice flour is best mixed with other flours as it has a strong flavour.

Sago flour is like rice flour in texture but comes from the trunk of the palm tree. It is almost pure starch with no strong flavour. It is good for making puddings and thickening stews.

Sorghum is a type of millet commonly eaten in Africa, North India and China. It is a good source of protein, calcium and iron. It may be used to make porridge or cooked as rice. The flour can be used in cakes or flatbreads.

Soya flour is made from ground soya beans. It is a good source of protein and B vitamins and is the only pulse to contain significant amounts of fat. It has a strong flavour and is best used in combination with other flours.

Tapioca comes from the root of the tropical plant, cassava. Like sago, it is almost pure starch. It can be used by itself to make a pudding, but it is also handy for thickening soups and stews. Cassava flour (or manioc) is usually coarser and may be blended with other flours to make bread.

Varieties of wheat

The following grains are all forms of wheat and are there-fore not suitable for an exclusion, gluten-free or wheat-free diet.

Bulgar is an ancient wheat that survived in Eastern Europe and is now eaten in many parts of the world. It is usually sold as cooked, parboiled wheat. It has a good taste and nutritional content.

Couscous is derived from semolina, which is a wheat product. A staple food of North Africa now readily available in Britain, it makes a good alternative to pasta, rice or potato.

Cracked wheat is made by splitting the hard outer casing of the grain. This retains its nutritional value while enabling it to cook faster.

Kibbled wheat is formed when the whole grain is cracked into little pieces rather than milled. It is used in bread-making and in breakfast cereals.

Semolina is a wheat product and should not be confused with short-grain rice, tapioca or sago.

Spelt and Kamut are ancient grains which have not been altered genetically over the years. Some people find they are able to tolerate these better than wheat, but they contain gluten and are not suitable for coeliacs.

Triticale is a man-made grain formed by crossing wheat and rye to improve nutritional value. It can be used to make bread.

Alternatives to dairy products

Soya milk is made from soya beans and may be obtained from health-food shops or supermarkets. Unopened, it does not need refrigeration, but after opening it should be kept in the refrigerator and used within three days. Soya milk can be used in cooking in the same way as cow's milk. Hot drinks should be allowed to cool slightly before adding soya milk to prevent it from separating. Soya milk is naturally low in calcium, but some brands are enriched with this mineral and are therefore a better substitute for cow's milk. These can be bought unsweetened, or sweetened with apple juice or fruit sugar.

There are a large number of useful soya products available, such as soya margarine, cheese, yoghurt, ice-creams and other desserts. These are all suitable for a milk-free diet but may contain ingredients not allowed on the exclusion diet and therefore labels should be checked carefully. Tofu is soya bean curd. It is high in protein and calcium and a good meat substitute for vegetarians. It is available plain or smoked. Plain varieties quickly absorb the flavour of a marinade and when stir-fried have a similar texture to chicken. Do not mistake Quorn for tofu. Quorn is made from a microfungus which is a relative of the mushroom and another good meat substitute. However, it contains egg white and is therefore not suitable for the initial stage of the exclusion diet.

Rice milks are also available in most health-food shops. They are made from brown rice and may have oil, salt and flavourings added. Nutritionally, they are not a good substitute for milk, but they are useful in expanding the diet if soya milk is not tolerated. *Oat milks* and *pea milks* are also now available.

Goat's and **sheep's milk**, cheese and yoghurt may be tested if cow's milk is not tolerated. However, they are similar in nature to cow's milk and should be avoided on the first stage of the exclusion diet. Some people with cow's milk intolerance find that after a while they also become intolerant of goat's and sheep's milk.

Spreading and cooking fats. Being a cow's milk product, butter is not allowed on exclusion and milk-free diets. Most margarines also contain milk and should be avoided. Margarines that are 100 per cent dairy-free include soya and sunflower varieties. They can be found in health-food shops and some supermarkets. Some varieties contain vegetable oils, which may or may not include corn (or maize) oil. This should be checked with the manufacturer (some addresses are given at the end of the book) to determine whether a margarine is suitable for the exclusion diet. Commercial vegetable oil is a blend of oils and usually contains corn. This should be avoided on the exclusion diet and replaced with, for example, sunflower, olive, rapeseed or safflower oils.

Egg substitutes. It is possible to replace eggs in recipes with commercial egg replacers. Although these have little nutritional value, they can be very useful in cooking. Check the ingredients carefully to determine whether they are suitable for the exclusion diet. Other substitutes for eggs in cooking are given in the introduction to the recipe section.

Alternative savoury flavourings

Miso is a fermented mixture of cereal grains, soya beans, water and salt. The form containing rice will be suitable for many people with food intolerance, but be careful not to confuse it with other varieties containing wheat or barley. Miso is rich in protein, minerals and vitamins, including vitamin B_{12}. It has a thick, pasty consistency and is thinned with water (but not boiling water, as this curdles it) to be used as a stock base in soups, stews, sauces and gravies.

Tahini is made from sesame seeds crushed and blended with oil. It is useful for making sauces and in the dip, hummus. For people who do not tolerate lemon, an added amount of garlic and parsley makes an excellent alternative. Tahini can also be included in salad dressing or spread on rice cakes.

Tamari is a wheat-free soy sauce. It is a useful flavouring in savoury dishes such as stir-fries and to enhance the flavour of gravy.

Gravy mixes usually contain yeast and wheat or corn starch. There are some gravy brownings available (e.g. Burdell's or Crosse and Blackwell's) that contain caramel and salt only and these can be added to meat juices to provide colour. Some health-food shops supply wheat- and yeast-free gravy mixes, but check the rest of the ingredients carefully.

Creamed coconut or **coconut milk** are useful ingredients, particularly in Chinese or Thai style dishes. They may be used in both savoury and sweet sauces.

Mirrin is a sweet Japanese seasoning, suitable for the exclusion diet. It is available from good health food shops and is useful in marinades and stir-fries. In some recipes it can be replaced with sweet rice vinegar.

Further suggestions for gravies, sauces and stocks are given in the relevant recipe section.

Alternative drinks

Cutting out tea and coffee offers a chance to experiment with a variety of alternative drinks. There is a wide range of herbal and fruit teas to choose from (avoid those with added citrus peel) as well as flavoured soya milks and fruit juices. Camomile tea or hot carob-flavoured soya milk are relaxing at bedtime. Use the carob flour like cocoa powder. Earlier in the day, peppermint tea or pineapple juice are refreshing. Rooibosh herbal tea is the closest in taste to normal tea. Chicory is a good alternative to coffee and the ground variety can be brewed in the same way as ground coffee. Soya milk shakes can be made at home by liquidizing fresh or tinned fruit with soya milk, or you can buy them from health-food shops. For a change, try a mixture of apple and grape juice with ice and a sprig of mint, or tomato juice with a touch of paprika.

The recipe section on beverages gives some more ideas for new drinks to try.

A sample menu

The simple guidelines below are intended to help make sure that the exclusion diet you are following is nutritionally balanced. You can exchange the foods listed with ideas from the relevant recipe sections in this book. For a main meal you may wish to add a soup or starter and in between meals you can try suggestions in the baking section. There are also recipe ideas for packed lunches and snacks, desserts and special occasions.

If you are hoping to lose weight on the exclusion diet, cut down on both fats and sugars. Do not fry foods, use only a scraping of margarine on rice cakes and do not use it on vegetables or add oily dressings to salads. Try to avoid sugary foods such as cakes and puddings; eat fresh fruit or fruit-based dishes instead.

If you are underweight, make desserts part of your meals and eat snacks in between. You should also have large portions of rice, sweet potatoes, meat and fish. Try to include plenty of soya products such as soya milk (as drinks and on cereal), soya yoghurt and other soya desserts.

Breakfast	Rice Krispies, soya milk and sugar
	Rice cakes, milk-free margarine and jam
	Apple juice/herbal tea
Snack meal	Meat/poultry/fish
	Cold rice salad or rice cakes
	Salad
	Fruit/soya yoghurt
	Ribena

Main meal	Meat/poultry/fish
	Sweet potato/rice/buckwheat pasta/rice noodles
	Vegetables
	Fruit- or soya-based dessert
	Herbal tea

Nutritional supplements

Vitamins and minerals

If your diet is varied and well balanced it is unlikely that you will need extra vitamins and minerals. If you are concerned that your diet is limited, ask your doctor to refer you to a state-registered dietitian who can recommend alternative foods rich in the nutrients you may be lacking or, if necessary, a suitable supplement. In some cases, individual vitamins or minerals may be necessary, e.g. calcium for those on a dairy-free diet.

If you are considering taking a supplement it is generally advisable to take a multivitamin or a multivitamin and mineral as a single tablet or capsule rather than large doses of individual vitamins and minerals. This is for several reasons:

- Water-soluble vitamins (vitamins B and C) are eliminated in the urine if they exceed the body's requirements. These vitamins are therefore wasted if taken in large doses.
- Some vitamins are toxic if taken in excessive quantities, e.g. vitamins A, D and B_6.
- Overdosing on single minerals may affect the absorption of others. Very high intakes of calcium or iron, for instance, can reduce absorption of zinc.
- Taking a combination of single, high dose minerals and vitamins is much more expensive than taking a single combined supplement.

Health supplements

There are a large number of 'health' supplements available that claim to ease a wide range of symptoms and ailments. However, few (if any) scientific trials have been performed to date to substantiate these claims. These supplements tend to be very expensive. If you wish to try a product but do not notice any improvement in your health after a few weeks, we suggest that you do not continue using it.

Prebiotics and probiotics

Recently there has been great interest by the public over probiotics. These are friendly bacteria that, it is hoped, may improve your health when taken regularly. Prebiotics are chemicals – usually special sorts of sugar – that will provide energy for probiotic bacteria to grow. Mixtures containing both probiotic bacteria and prebiotic sugars are sometimes available and have been called synbiotics.

We all know that there are billions and billions of bacteria and fungi (yeasts) living in the human intestine. Most of these are found in the large intestine, where they perform important functions. They not only break down dangerous chemicals but also synthesize vitamins and other substances, such as amino-acids and short-chain fatty acids, that are absorbed into the body to improve nutrition. Although the importance of infection by pathogenic (disease-causing) bacteria is well known, such as Salmonella or Campylobacter, which may both cause food poisoning, there is now increasing interest in the possibility that upsets in the healthy bacteria of the bowel could be a factor causing chronic diseases, even when no pathogenic bacteria can be detected.

Nearly 100 years ago, doctors noticed that some people in Bulgaria and other central European countries lived to a great age – sometimes as much as 120. They discovered that these people often drank sour milk and ate yoghurts, suggesting that the bacteria contained in these foods might be beneficial. It is only fairly recently that this idea has taken root in Western Europe, but now a bewildering array of these probiotic bacteria is available in every supermarket and health-food shop. It has even been suggested in television advertisements that to stay healthy one should occasionally 'top up' one's bowel bacteria by taking some of these preparations of probiotic bacteria. Are probiotic bacteria as helpful as is claimed?

Most probiotic bacteria available on sale are derived from those used in the manufacture of yoghurts and sour milks. They are usually Lactobacilli and/or Bifidobacteria, and both these types can be used for the manufacture of yoghurt. Many 'bio' yoghurts contain live bacteria added after the fermentation process is complete. Some other types of bacteria and yeasts are also available, but these are not as frequently used. Lactobacilli and Bifidobacteria also live in the normal healthy human intestine, and it has been found that their numbers are reduced in people suffering from certain disorders, in particular irritable bowel syndrome and Crohn's disease.

It would seem logical, therefore, to give probiotic bacteria to patients with these conditions in the hope that they might bring about an improvement, or even cure the disease. Unfortunately, although some benefit has been reported in some trials, most studies have been disappointing. Although probably hundreds of probiotic bacterial strains are now available for sale, none has proved so effective that it is licensed for prescription by the National Health Service. What is the reason for this apparent paradox?

In the first instance, it must be realised that the bacteria living in our intestines provide one of our most important defences against infection. We are all exposed each day to a steady stream of foreign bacteria, in our food, on things that we handle, and in the atmosphere. Some of these are pathogens. Any that are swallowed and survive, after passing through the strong acid of the stomach, find great difficulty in finding somewhere in the intestine to lodge and grow. The strong digestive enzymes of the small intestine prevent most bacteria from surviving there. In the large intestine, there is competition with the resident bacteria, which are already deeply entrenched. In addition, foreign bacteria come under attack from the immune system. These factors are collectively known as Colonization Resistance.

When we are born, our intestinal tracts are sterile, and no bacteria exist within them. It is crucial for the healthy growth of the child that a bacterial population is established in the gut, as this enables the development of an effective immune system, without which the child's defences against infectious diseases would be dangerously weak. Most of the bacteria that colonize the gut come from the mother, starting with the very process of birth, but continuing until the baby is two or three months old. During this time the baby has no immune system of its own and relies for protection on antibodies received from its mother in the womb or passed on during breast feeding.

The baby is at this time tolerant to antigens (disease 'particles') coming from outside the body, and cannot attack them. After two to three months, when the gut flora is established, this tolerance disappears and for the rest of its life the child's immune system will attack any substance entering the body that it does not recognise as part of its own make-up – and this includes new bacteria. It seems likely that the reason for the immune tolerance that exists in young infants is that it allows the development of a healthy variety of bacteria living in the gut. It would logically follow, however, that when immune tolerance disappears, the child has to live thereafter with those bacteria to which it has already been exposed, and that all new ones, be they harmless or pathogen, will be rejected.

This presents considerable advantages in the face of dangerous pathogenic bacteria, which will be quickly attacked and prevented from invading the body. On the other hand it means that friendly probiotic bacteria are unlikely to be able to become established, except perhaps under very special circumstances. Studies in which probiotic bacteria have been given to patients reveal that while the organisms can be found in the faeces during the feeding period, they rapidly disappear once feeding of the probiotic is stopped. Of course, if the bacteria in a probiotic mixture contained the very same strain as one which was missing from your gut, then this would survive and multiply, and there would be rapid and permanent improvement in your condition. However, given the number of strains of Lactobacilli and Bifidobacteria that exist, the chances of this happening is small.

Thus it is not easy, at present, to top up one's gut bacteria, or to introduce a new healthy strain. It might be hoped that feeding prebiotics, to increase the numbers of bacteria already present, might be more successful, but when we tried this in a study of irritable bowel syndrome we had no success.

Is there any point at all, then, in taking probiotics? The answer is that sometimes they may prove useful. During the time the probiotic bacteria are passing through the gut, they may exert a beneficial effect that will rapidly cease when feeding is stopped. In some patients with irritable bowel syndrome or Crohn's disease, this may provide some relief from symptoms, or allow foods to be eaten that usually cause problems. It is important that any probiotic preparation tried contains large numbers of living bacteria – ideally more than 10 billion per gram – and the greater the number of different types of bacteria present in the mixture, the better the chances that a useful metabolic effect will occur. A preparation – pill, drink or yoghurt – containing a single organism is unlikely to be as effective. There is no point in continuing with a probiotic mixture if you do not find benefit in the first two weeks.

Crohn's Disease

Introduction

Crohn's disease is a serious inflammatory condition that can affect any part of the gut, from mouth to anus, but which most frequently attacks the lower small bowel or the large intestine. It is usually treated with drugs, as discussed below, and, if necessary, surgery, but unfortunately these are not cures. It is, however, possible to treat Crohn's disease successfully with diet as there is evidence that the inflammation is associated with food intolerance. Dietary treatment of Crohn's disease is a complex procedure that may take several months to complete. Therefore, as Crohn's is a potentially dangerous condition if not properly controlled, **it is essential that all dietary studies are carried out with the knowledge and support of your specialist, GP and the hospital dietetic team.** Indeed, dietary treatment must be started by taking pre-digested elemental feeds, which are available only on prescription.

The cause of Crohn's disease is not yet understood, and there is no specific treatment. It is known that there is an inflammatory attack by the body's immune defences against the friendly bacteria that live in the intestines. The reason for this development is still unclear, but current treatment is designed to block the inflammatory process using drugs, such as corticosteroids ('steroids'), which suppress the immune system, or to use antibiotics to reduce the activity of the gut bacteria. Unfortunately, neither of these approaches is very effective. In general, only 50–60 per cent of patients will respond to a specific medication. In addition, patients may develop dangerous side effects to any of these drugs. Corticosteroids, for example, have multiple side effects, including thinning of the bones, high blood pressure, weight gain and diabetes. Other immunosuppressant drugs, such as azathioprine, may cause side effects such as damage to the bone marrow in as many as 20 per cent of patients. Infliximab, a newly available antibody treatment, may cause re-activation of tuberculosis in patients with a history of this infection. If drug treatment fails and the bowel becomes badly damaged or obstructed, the patient will require surgery.

So why diet?

Patients with Crohn's disease frequently lose weight and become malnourished. It was the introduction of intravenous feeding – that is, feeding through a vein rather than by mouth – to combat malnutrition that lead to the discovery of dietary treatment. Patients who required surgery were often so poorly nourished that their operations had to be delayed until this could be corrected. It was found that patients fed intravenously not only gained weight, but also reported that their symptoms of diarrhoea and pain improved. When they returned to normal eating, however, they rapidly relapsed.

Intravenous feeding is potentially dangerous because of the risks, especially of infection. It was soon discovered, however, that elemental feeds were just as effective as intravenous nutrition in relieving the symptoms of Crohn's disease. Elemental feeds had been developed by NASA for use by astronauts. They were pre-digested liquid foods whose contents were broken down to their simplest components – proteins to amino acids and starches to sugars – with a single fatty oil, minerals and vitamins being added to make them nutritionally adequate. Despite flavourings, they tasted dreadful at first. Nowadays the flavour is much improved and the majority of patients can drink elemental feeds without great difficulty.

Elemental feeds are highly effective in relieving Crohn's disease. As many as 80–90 per cent of patients who are willing to stick to an elemental diet will find that their symptoms clear in two to three weeks. Such a time away from normal eating obviously demands great determination, but the improvement of symptoms provides a strong incentive for the patient to continue.

How does dietary treatment work?

There is still disagreement as to how an elemental diet works in Crohn's disease. It was initially suggested that it might allow the gut to rest, or that it improved nutrition, or that it removed food allergens from the diet. We now know that all these are only partially true, if at all. We believe that an elemental diet is effective because it deprives the bowel bacteria of the energy they require to thrive. An elemental diet is quickly and completely absorbed in the upper small intestine and little, if any, residue passes down to the lower gut where most bacteria live. After one week of elemental feeding, the number of bacteria falls by more than half, and their activity is reduced. This results in a decline in the immune attack on the bacteria, and so the disease improves.

When the patient's symptoms have settled, the elemental diet may be stopped. However, returning to a normal diet will lead to a rapid relapse. The next stage in treatment, therefore, involves the gradual reintroduction of normal foods in a carefully controlled manner so that any that provoke symptoms are identified and thereafter avoided. We believe that specific foods stimulate bacterial activity and hence reactivate the disease. Unfortunately these foods may differ from patient to patient. In coeliac disease, 97 per cent of patients respond successfully to a gluten-free diet, and treatment is therefore relatively simple. In Crohn's disease, there is a range of foods that may be implicated. One patient may be upset by chocolate and peanuts, for example, and another by wheat and milk. Likewise, the number of problem foods concerned may vary, from a single item to as many as a dozen. The process of food reintroduction is therefore crucial to the success of the procedure, and should be undertaken with the regular support and supervision of a state-registered dietitian.

The simplest way of reintroducing food into the diet is to start on an exclusion diet, similar to that used for irritable bowel syndrome. This is a balanced diet, avoiding those foods most frequently reported by Crohn's sufferers to cause upset. Foods that are high in fat and fibre also commonly cause problems for Crohn's patients and so these too are limited in the initial stages of the diet. The diet that we have developed is thus known as a LOw Fat, Fibre Limited EXclusion diet, usually referred to as LOFFLEX. This allows the patient to switch straight from the elemental diet to a range of foods that rarely cause difficulties. If after a further two weeks he or she is still feeling well, then the remaining foods are reintroduced slowly and carefully in order to detect intolerances. The LOFFLEX diet is also sometimes helpful for patients with rheumatoid arthritis (see page 11).

If problems arise on the LOFFLEX diet, it is necessary to follow an elimination diet – a slower and more cumbersome procedure. Here, a single new food is reintroduced every day while continuing on the elemental feeds, until there are sufficient normal foods to allow a balanced diet. This may be a more successful method of reintroduction for a patient with unusual food intolerances. Full practical details of these diets will be given later (page 63). When the food reintroductions are complete, it is necessary for the dietitian to check the final diet to ensure that it is nutritionally adequate, and to suggest ways of correcting any deficiencies.

Understandably, a number of patients fail to complete such a demanding dietary programme. In our experience 25–30 per cent are unable to continue on an elemental diet long enough to reach remission. A further 10–15 per cent drop out during the process of food reintroduction. However, once food intolerances have been accurately established, relapse is unusual if the patient keeps to the diet. We have found that nearly 60 per cent of patients are still well two years after starting the diet, with no other treatment required. It is most unusual for these patients subsequently to relapse, and after five years, many find that they can slowly return to normal eating, as the Crohn's disease appears to burn itself out. There are few if any side effects. We have shown that these patients do not develop thinning of the bones, and women can undergo normal pregnancies without changing their treatment. Perhaps most important of all, the patient feels in complete control of the Crohn's disease, and is able to ensure that it does not cause difficulties at crucial moments, such as exams or holidays.

In Crohn's disease, diet is effective only against active inflammation. It will not correct infection, previous damage to the bowel, or the effects of surgery. There is no point in starting the diet if the disease is inactive. It is most important to check with your doctors that inflammation is the likely cause of your symptoms before setting out to try dietary treatment. Diet is not an effective treatment for ulcerative colitis.

Stage 1: Achieving remission on the elemental diet

If your doctor agrees that diet is an appropriate treatment for your active Crohn's disease, you will need to start off with a course of elemental feeds. This can only be obtained with a prescription from your doctor. Dietary treatment will not be effective if you are on a high dose of corticosteroids and you will need to discuss with your doctor how gradually to reduce your medication before starting, or while you are taking, elemental feeds. **Do not change any medication without your doctor's advice.** This could potentially be very dangerous, especially if you are taking a corticosteroid. This is a type of hormone that your body normally produces, but in smaller amounts. When you are taking these pills, your body adapts to this supply and stops making the hormone itself. If you suddenly stop taking the medication, your body will not have time to turn on its own supplies again, leading to a hormone deficiency that can be very dangerous.

Your doctor will refer you to a dietitian, who will advise you on how to take the elemental feeds. The dietitian will explain how much you will need to drink each day so as to reach or maintain a healthy weight. For the diet to succeed all other foods and drinks, apart from water, must be stopped. In our experience, Elemental 028 Extra (SHS International Ltd) is very effective. This is available in a liquid or powder form. The liquid form is supplied in a 250 ml 'Tetra-pak', currently with a choice of three flavours. The powdered from can be obtained pre-flavoured, or unflavoured and with a choice of seven flavour sachets that you can add. It should be reconstituted with water and chilled.

The elemental diet needs to be introduced slowly over a few days, gradually building up to the quantity recommended by your dietitian. It is best to sip the feed slowly throughout the day, rather than taking it only at mealtimes. The feed tastes better when chilled; some people like to eat it semi-frozen as a fruit slush. You may develop headaches during the first few days as your body gets used to the drink. This can be particularly noticeable if you are used to drinking a lot of tea or coffee and suffer caffeine withdrawal, but the headaches should soon pass. Make sure you drink plenty of water, particularly in the early stages when you are building up the volume of elemental diet.

Some people feel nauseous at the start of treatment. Drinking through a straw or diluting the feed with a little more water can help. However, do not dilute it so much that you struggle to consume the volume of elemental diet you need each day. You will probably notice that your stools turn green and that you develop bad breath. Don't worry. These are both normal effects of the elemental diet and show that it is working by blocking the activities of your bowel bacteria. Brushing your teeth more regularly will help improve your breath, and these effects will soon clear when you get back to eating ordinary foods again.

Usually symptoms have improved by around seven days but it is essential that you complete the prescribed course, in order to get the underlying inflammation properly under control. This usually takes between two and three weeks, although your doctor may advise you to continue for a little longer if your symptoms have not entirely settled at the end of this period. There is no point in starting the next stage of treatment if your disease is still active.

Stage 2: Reintroducing and testing foods

By now you should be feeling very much better and longing to eat again. However, returning to a normal diet now will take you straight back to square one. To maintain remission from the disease, you must find out which foods are safe for you to eat and which are not. This can only be done by testing foods individually to see which ones cause your symptoms to return. However, testing every single food would take a very long time. Having treated many patients with Crohn's disease, we have found that there are a number of foods that rarely cause problems and therefore can be reintroduced into the diet straight away. These foods form the basis of the diet.

Fatty foods and high fibre foods often upset Crohn's disease. As the liquid elemental diet is fibre-free and low in fat, it seems sensible to start on an exclusion diet with a reduced fat and fibre content, and to increase these gradually to the individual's level of tolerance. For this reason, the exclusion diet we recommend for Crohn's disease is known as the LOFFLEX diet. It is similar to that used in irritable bowel syndrome, but the foods concerned are slightly different. Potato, for example, is sometimes a problem in irritable bowel syndrome but rarely in Crohn's disease. The foods that are allowed and those that must be avoided are shown below.

The LOFFLEX diet

	Not allowed	Allowed
Meat	Pork, ham, bacon, meat products, e.g. sausages, beefburgers, meat pies, pâté and meat paste	All other lean meat and poultry, e.g. lean beef, lamb, chicken (avoid skin and visible fat)
Fish	Fish in batter, crumb, or tinned in oil or tomato, fish paste, taramasalata, scampi	White fish, tinned tuna in oil, small portions of fatty, smoked and other tinned fish (in water or brine), shellfish
Vegetables	Pulses (peas, beans, lentils), onions, sweet-corn, tomatoes (including ketchup and purée), tinned vegetables in sauce, e.g. baked beans	Small portions of all other vegetables, without skins, seeds or stalks, maximum two portions per day
Fruit	Citrus fruit, e.g. oranges, lemons, satsumas, grapefruit. Apples, bananas, dried fruit, marmalade	Small portions of all other fruits, without skin or seeds, maximum two portions per day, fresh, or cooked. Jams free of orange/apple
Cereals	Wheat, oats, rye, corn, barley (see pages 262–265 for foods containing these)	White rice, rice pasta, rice cakes, puffed rice cereal, rice flour, ground rice, tapioca, sago, arrowroot
Cooking oils	Corn oil, vegetable oil, nut oils	Sunflower, soya, olive, rape-seed oils (use sparingly, stir-fry only)
Dairy products	Cow's, goat's, sheep's milk and products, e.g. butter, margarine, cream, yoghurt,	Soya milk and products, e.g. dairy-free margarine, soya yoghurt, soya cream and soya ice-cream (small

	Not allowed	Allowed
	ice-cream, cheese, eggs (see pages 261–262 for foods containing these)	portions only as high in fat), tofu
Beverages	Tea, coffee (including decaffeinated), fruit squashes and fizzy drinks, citrus, apple and tomato juice, all types of alcohol	Tap or mineral water, herbal and fruit teas (not containing citrus fruit or apple), other fruit juice, e.g. pineapple, grape, blackcurrant
Miscellaneous	Yeast (see page 264 for foods containing this), salad cream and dress-ings, mustard, soy sauce, tinned and packet sauces (see recipe section for alternatives), nuts, seeds, chocolate	Salt, pepper, herbs, spices (in moderation), vinegar, sugar, honey, syrup, Kendal mint cake, carob

Following the LOFFLEX diet

Here are some guidelines to help you follow the diet:

1. Try to eat a wide variety of foods in the allowed list to help keep your diet balanced and interesting. You may find the sample menu below helpful. If you are struggling to find foods that you like, discuss this with your dietitian, who may be able to suggest alternatives.

Breakfast	Rice cereal, soya milk and sugar Rice cakes, milk-free margarine and honey, herbal tea
Snack meal	Lean red meat *or* fish *or* chicken/turkey Jacket potato (no skin) *or* rice *or* rice cakes

	Small portion of salad Piece of fruit (from allowed list)
Main meal	Lean meat *or* fish *or* chicken/turkey Potato *or* rice *or* rice pasta Cooked vegetables *or* salad (small portion from allowed list) Soya milk-based dessert and portion of fruit (from allowed list)

2. Throughout the diet, keep a record of everything you eat and drink, and any symptoms you experience (similar to the food and symptom diary shown on page 34 for the exclusion diet). This will help make it easier to identify any foods that you are intolerant to, even among those that are normally found to be safe.

3. Keep in regular contact with your dietitian to discuss your progress. If you feel your symptoms are beginning to return, it is essential that you report this as soon as possible. Be honest with your dietitian; if you are finding it a struggle sticking to the diet, let him or her know – a regular phone call should help to keep you motivated.

4. If all remains well after two weeks, your doctor and dietitian may feel you are ready to start reintroducing other foods into the diet. **Do not start to do this until you have been given the go-ahead.** Sometimes, another week or two on the basic diet may be of benefit.

Reintroducing foods

Follow the instructions for reintroducing foods as given in the section on the exclusion diet for irritable bowel syndrome (pages 31–43). However, there are some important differences in Crohn's disease:

- Each food should be tested for *four* days (and wheat for *seven* days). Include the test food at two separate meals or snacks each day, or as indicated in the list below. If there is no reaction, the food can be kept in the diet and eaten in normal quantities.

- If you react to a food, stop testing immediately. Do not continue testing for the full four days as this may cause your condition to relapse. Contact your dietitian and delay any further testing until you are fully recovered.

- If you have a particularly bad reaction to a food, you may need to have a short course of elemental diet to settle your symptoms. You must discuss this with your dietitian and/or doctor, who will arrange a prescription for more elemental feeds if you have run out. When you are ready to return to testing you do not need to start all over again from the beginning. Simply return to where you were in the list of reintroductions before you suffered the adverse reaction, obviously, avoiding the problematic food.

- Foods that are high in fibre (e.g. oats, rye, banana, peas, wholegrain wheat, nuts, sweetcorn and barley) should be consumed in small portions on the first day, gradually increasing portion sizes over the remaining three days. If you notice an increase in discomfort or flatulence, or your stools become looser, return to smaller portion sizes. If symptoms do not settle straight away, cut those foods out and test again at a later date with small portion sizes. Testing high-fibre foods this way will help you to discover whether the return of your symptoms is due to an intolerance to the food itself or to the amount of fibre it contains. It should help you to determine a suitable level of fibre in your diet.

- Similarly, foods that are high in fat (e.g. butter, margarine, chocolate, cheese) should be eaten in small amounts to begin with and then gradually increased, as tolerated.

Order of food reintroduction

The order of reintroductions on the LOFFLEX diet is as
follows:

Pork	– test as ham or bacon for snack meal, and as roast, chop or mince for main meal
Oats	– test porridge, oatcakes, flapjacks (check other ingredients)
Tea	– at least twice per day
Ryvita	– test at two meals per day
Eggs	– test at two meals per day
Onions	– test cooked and raw
Coffee	– test instant and coffee beans
Yeast	– take three brewers' yeast tablets (one with each meal), available from pharmacies
Banana	– test two per day
Apple	– as for banana
Milk	– test 560 ml–1 pint spread over the day
Butter or margarine	– test at all three meals
White wine	– test two glasses per day. If okay, try red wine. If yeast is not tolerated, try spirits
Peas	– test at two meals per day, if possible
Chocolate	– test as plain chocolate, if milk not tolerated, or as cocoa
Tomatoes	– test cooked and raw
Cheese	– test cooked and raw
Corn	– test corn flakes or cornflour in cooking
Citrus fruit	– test oranges, grapefruit, satsumas etc, or as fruit juice
Wheat	– test for seven days, taking wheat at each meal. See page 36 on how to test wheat
Yoghurt	– at two meals per day, natural or flavoured
Nuts	– try different varieties, 60 g/2 oz per day
Sweetcorn	– small portions initially, as very high in fibre
Barley	– test barley flakes and pearl barley

- When testing foods, it is important to remember that any unpleasant symptoms may indicate a reaction – it is not always the case that stomach pains or diarrhoea are the first symptoms to appear. During the period of food reintroduction, it should be assumed that all symptoms are caused by the food in question. However, symptoms may arise in other ways – e.g. during the menstrual cycle – and thus complicate the procedure. For this reason it is necessary to re-test all foods that seem to trigger problems to make certain they really are the cause of the trouble. Leave two- or three-week gaps before re-testing a food that may have upset you, as repeatedly retrying a single food slows your progress considerably and tends to reduce morale.

- When you have completed all the testing, your dietitian will need to assess the nutritional adequacy of your final diet. You may be asked to complete an accurate diary of everything you eat and drink for a week. Analysis of your diary will indicate whether your diet is low in any of the essential nutrients. The dietitian can advise you on which foods you could increase to improve the nutritional balance. It may also be necessary to supplement your diet with minerals or vitamins. **It is an essential part of dietary treatment that your final diet is checked by a state-registered dietitian.**

The elimination diet

Occasionally, patients may find that their disease goes into remission while on the elemental diet but as soon as they start the LOFFLEX diet, they relapse straight away. This may be due to an undetected narrowing of the gut due to strictures. In this case the liquid diet will pass through without problem but any solid food will cause discomfort. Or it may indicate that a patient is intolerant to one or more of the 'safe' foods on the basic LOFFLEX diet. If further investigations rule out the presence of strictures, the patient can proceed with dietary treatment by introducing foods in a different way – known as the elimination diet.

The elimination diet does not presume that any food is safe. Therefore, all foods have to be tested. This is obviously a more time-consuming approach and requires a patient to continue with elemental feeds until enough different foods have been reintroduced for the diet to be nutritionally balanced. Because the list of foods to be tested is so long, the testing period for each food is normally one day only. This can turn out to be too short, as some food reactions come on quite slowly. Therefore it is sometimes better to slow the process of food testing. This is particularly important when testing cereal grains, and, as with the LOFFLEX diet, it is recommended that wheat is tested for seven days.

As with LOFFLEX, it is essential that patients on the elimination diet are in regular contact with their dietitian and that they keep a detailed food and symptom diary throughout. During the first two weeks, the elemental diet can be gradually reduced, with the guidance of the dietitian. Foods being tested should be eaten at least twice that day and if no symptoms are experienced, can thereafter be taken in normal quantities in the diet. Foods that cause a reaction should be stopped immediately and further testing suspended until the patient is fully recovered. This may sometimes take several days. As with the LOFFLEX diet, elemental feeds may be required for a day or two to settle a particularly bad reaction.

The first few days of food reintroductions are normally as follows:

Day 1	Chicken
Day 2	Rice
Day 3	Pears
Day 4	Soya margarine

Day 5	Soya milk
Day 6	Carrots
Day 7	Potatoes
Days 8–9	No further testing, continue on safe foods
Day 10	White fish
Day 11	Runner beans
Day 12	Cooking oil
Day 13	Bananas
Day 14	Turkey
Day 15	Peas
Day 16	Milk
Days 17–18	No further testing, continue on safe foods

Continue to introduce foods each day, taking three to four days to test oats, corn, rye and barley, and seven days to test wheat. As in the LOFFLEX diet, gradually increase portion sizes of high-fibre cereals, vegetables and fruits to determine the level of fibre that is tolerated. When testing foods, it is important to remember that any unpleasant symptoms may indicate a reaction – it is not always the case that stomach pains or diarrhoea are the first symptoms to appear. During the period of food reintroduction, it should be assumed that all symptoms are caused by the food in question. Final diets must be assessed in the same way as the LOFFLEX to check that they are nutritionally adequate.

Keeping well on your diet

It is important to remember that the diet you are following is an active treatment for a potentially dangerous disease, and it must be continued if you wish to avoid a relapse. It is not possible to take a 'diet holiday'. Many feel so well on their diets that they are tempted to believe that the Crohn's disease has gone, and that they will be able to eat anything they like. This is sadly not true. You may find that you get away with eating a problem food once, or even twice, but if you continue to eat it the disease will recur after a few days. Most patients find that five to ten years elapse before they can be really confident that problem foods no longer upset them. It is reasonable to re-test foods every year to make sure that they still cause trouble.

Sometimes it is difficult when travelling or visiting friends to avoid eating something that you know upsets you. If this happens, try to keep strictly to your diet for several days afterwards to allow the effects of this food to pass away. It is sensible always to have a small supply of elemental feed available, in case of bad reactions, or if you get a gut upset, perhaps from food poisoning or antibiotics. This will help prevent these setbacks developing into full relapses. When the symptoms subside, you will be able to go straight back to your previous diet.

Patients who control their Crohn's disease successfully through diet are delighted with their progress. Although diet may sound daunting, it is well worth the effort.

The Recipes

Introduction

An exclusion diet need not be repetitive and boring. Many of the recipes in the following sections were designed by Pamela Harris, who has been on a restricted diet herself for 14 years. Through her research she has gained a wealth of experience in creating delicious dishes. She has broadcast on radio on the subject of alternative foods, as well as giving advice to children and adults about food intolerance. She also writes for a monthly publication for children.

Cooking with unfamiliar foods may appear daunting at first, but with patience and practice you may well be surprised with the results. These tips from Pamela should help make your new style of cooking both enjoyable and successful:

- If you are unable to find an ingredient that appears in these recipes in your local supermarket or health food shop, check the specialist suppliers (see pages 273–275) for availability. Chinese and Indian supermarkets and delicatessens are also good places to look and are often much cheaper. Buy a small amount initially, but if you find the products useful, order in bulk later to save money. The same ingredients have been used in a number of different recipes to minimize any waste.

- Try to build up some store-cupboard ingredients, such as:

rice noodles	pumpkin seeds	banana chips
ground rice	sunflower seeds	dried apricots
arrowroot	pine nuts (not true nuts)	dried mango
pulses and beans	desiccated coconut	dried pineapple
spices		

- Buy fresh herbs in pots and use over two to three days. Continue to water the pot and you should get a second growth. Put any leftovers in the freezer. Herb oils are excellent and have a long shelf life. Buy a large bottle of your supermarket's own brand of sunflower oil. Decant into smaller bottles and add plenty of herbs, for example, lemon thyme or marjoram. Seal the bottles and let them stand for at least a month before using.

- Keep all alternative flours in the refrigerator to prolong their freshness.

- When making bread, make two loaves at a time and keep spare slices and a bag of breadcrumbs in the freezer. A bag of frozen home-made cake crumbs is also very useful.

- Wheat-free flours are lighter than normal flour and therefore less fat is needed than in standard recipes.

- Wheat-free products require a lower temperature and a longer cooking time. Refrigerating the dough for 20–30 minutes before baking helps improve the flavour and texture. Use smaller dishes and tins, greasing them very well.

- Home-made stock has the best flavour and is the most economical (see page 190). Buy cheap offcuts of meat from your butcher and boil them with vegetables and herbs to make a stock. If cooking for one or two people, freeze it in an ice-cube tray. For convenience, you can also use some of the commercial products that are available. Supermarkets offer their own fresh stocks, although chicken stock tends to be the only one suitable for the exclusion diet (check the ingredients carefully). Some stock cubes and powders available from health food shops are wheat-, dairy- and yeast-free.

• When buying meat, especially cubed, look in supermarket freezer cabinets, which stock lean, economically priced packs of beef, lamb, pork and chicken.

• Sugar in recipes can be replaced with honey or a concentrated syrupy fruit juice. However, remember that these contain more moisture and you may not need to add as much liquid as the recipe suggests. Fruit sugar, or fructose, may also be used in place of sugar. In general, reduce the amount in the recipe by a quarter.

• Soya cream works well in recipes and is reasonably heat stable. Check ingredients are suitable for your diet.

• Check when buying spices that these are wheat-free.

• In most pasta dishes, pasta can be replaced with rice or rice noodles.

• For those who have problems with eggs, here are some tips:

Use unflavoured vegetable gelatine instead (1 tsp dry gelatine to 2 tbsp liquid for each egg).
Substitute mashed banana, apricot purée or puréed vegetables (2 tbsp for each egg).
Various egg replacers are on the market. Check carefully, as most contain whey powder.

- Electrical kitchen equipment, e.g. blenders, liquidizers and food processors, make life a lot easier. You will need to add less liquid using this equipment than if you are mixing by hand. Add liquid gradually to prevent the mixture from becoming too heavy – you will learn to find the right consistency through experience.

- Finally, do not expect too much too quickly. Read as much as you can about the ingredients you are using and scan cookery books for ideas. You will soon find you can select information that relates to you and customize recipes to suit your requirements.

Symbols

The recipes in this book are, as far as possible, free from artificial colourings, flavourings and preservatives. They are also free from gluten (wheat, rye and barley), wheat starch, oats, cow's milk and corn (apart from some of the flour mixes used in the baking section). If you are following the first stage of the exclusion diet, the LOFFLEX diet or are excluding eggs you should select only those appropriately marked (see below). If other foods are to be excluded you will need to examine the list of ingredients in each recipe carefully to see whether it is suitable for your diet. Check labels carefully for ingredients such as wheat-free mustard, worcester sauce and curry powder. These vary between manufacturers and may or may not be suitable for the exclusion and LOFFLEX diets.

The symbols used in this book for the special diets are:

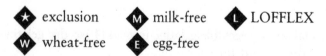

◆ exclusion   ◆ milk-free   ◆ LOFFLEX
◆ wheat-free   ◆ egg-free

Measurements

Often measurements are given in both metric and imperial units. Use one system only; do not combine them.

Where spoonfuls are referred to, level spoons are meant unless otherwise stated.

1 tsp (teaspoon) = 5 ml
1 tbsp (tablespoon) = 15 ml
1 tbsp = 3 tsp

To ensure success, check the size of the spoons you are using. Australian readers should remember that since their tablespoon has been converted to 20 ml, it is larger than the British tablespoon. They must therefore use three 5 ml teaspoons wherever the recipes demand a tablespoon.

Oven temperatures

As different makes of oven vary so much, it is necessary to know your own oven or to keep an oven thermometer permanently in the oven. Below is a chart outlining oven temperatures. Any baking recipe including wheat-free flour mixes should always be cooked at a lower temperature and for a longer time than one using wheat flour: a high temperature can release fats from the ingredients which would make baking oily and some dishes unsuccessful. Cooking with alternative ingredients does take practice but with a little patience you will achieve a culinary expertise that will mean you can cook when entertaining guests and they will be unaware of any difference.

°C	°F	Gas Mark	Description
110	225	¼	Very slow
120	250	½	Very slow
140	275	1	Slow
150	300	2	Slow
160	325	3	Moderate
180	350	4	Moderate
190	375	5	Moderately hot
200	400	6	Moderately hot
220	425	7	Hot
230	450	8	Hot
240	475	9	Very hot

Breakfasts

Breakfast cheers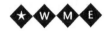

Serves 1

1 small tub soya yoghurt
1 dessertspoon clear honey
6 dried apricots, poached, plus 1–2 tbsp of the poaching juice

Put all the ingredients into a blender and process to a smooth drink, adding a little more apricot juice if necessary. Raspberries can be used in place of apricots to vary the flavour.

Breakfast crunch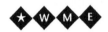

Serves 2

1 small tub soya yoghurt
1 tsp clear honey
1 tbsp sunflower seeds, toasted
1 tsp raisins, chopped
1 tsp dried apricots, chopped

Empty the yoghurt into a sundae dish and drizzle with the honey. Mix together the seeds, raisins and apricots and sprinkle on top.

Winter warmer breakfast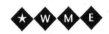

Serves 2

60 g/2 oz mixture of rice and millet flakes
200 ml/⅓ pint water
2 tsp clear honey (to taste)
1 level tbsp dried apricots
1 level tbsp mixture of sultanas, raisins or chopped dates

Put the flakes and water in a saucepan, bring to the boil and simmer for 3–4 minutes. Remove from the heat and stir in the honey, apricots and other fruit of choice.

Pan-fried herring roes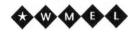

Serves 1

115 g/4 oz herring roes
30 g/1 oz dairy-free margarine plus 1 tsp sunflower oil
little rice vinegar
salt and pepper

Put the roes in a basin, cover with water and add 1 dessert-spoon of rice vinegar. Leave for 10 minutes to clean. Drain and rinse the roes in fresh cold water and pat dry.

Put the oil and margarine in a shallow pan and heat gently; do not allow the margarine to brown. Lay the roes in the pan, season and cook gently for about 6–7 minutes, depending on thickness, turning once.

Remove the roes, drain on kitchen paper and transfer to a plate. Keep warm.

If necessary, add a little fresh margarine to the juices in pan. Add 1 tsp rice vinegar (or to taste). Add parsley and stir together. Spoon the juices over the roes and serve.

Zingy mushrooms

Serves 1

2 large flat mushrooms
1 heaped tbsp rice, preferably brown, cooked
1 medium tomato, skinned and chopped
1 tsp wheat-free Worcester sauce, or to taste
½ tbsp wheat-free mustard
small knob dairy-free margarine
salt and pepper

Wipe the mushrooms clean. Mix together the rice and tomato, season lightly and add the Worcester sauce and mustard. Mix well.

Spread the mixture over the mushrooms and dot the top with a small knob of margarine.

Bake at 180°C/350°F/Gas Mark 4 for 15–20 minutes.

Bacon rosti brunch

Serves 1

115 g/4 oz unsmoked streaky bacon, de-rinded and chopped
115 g/4 oz sweet potatoes, coarsely grated
115 g/4 oz cabbage, finely shredded
1 egg, beaten
1 tsp rice or millet flour mix
2 spikes chives, chopped
salt and pepper

Put the bacon, potatoes and cabbage in a bowl and season to taste. Stir in the flour and chives, add the egg and mix well.

Heat a little oil in frying pan, drop in spoonfuls of mixture, and fry for about 7–8 minutes, turning once.

Drain on kitchen paper and serve with grilled tomatoes.

Pear to please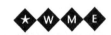

Serves 1

1 large fresh pear
1 heaped tbsp ready-to-eat prunes, minced
1 tbsp pure apricot preserve
toasted pine nuts (optional)

Peel and halve the pear, gently removing the core. Mix the prunes with the apricot preserve and fill the pear. Sprinkle with the toasted pine nuts if desired.

Honeyed banana bread

Serves 1

2 slices wheat-free bread (see page 214)
1 banana
1 tbsp clear honey, warmed
pinch cinnamon

Wrap the bread slices loosely in tin foil. Put in the oven to slightly warm through. Remove from the oven and place on a warm plate.

Mash the banana and add the warm honey. Spread over the slices of bread and lightly dust with cinnamon.

Raisin start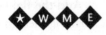

Serves 2

5 g/3 oz seedless raisins
2 ripe pears
1 small tub soya yoghurt
little cinnamon (to taste)

Soak the raisins in just enough hot water to cover for 15–20 minutes, until plump and moist. Meanwhile, peel and core the pears and cut into chunks.

Put the yoghurt in a blender, drain the raisins and add to the blender along with the pears. Blend together until fairly smooth.

Pour into individual dishes and sprinkle with cinnamon to taste.

Tropical muesli

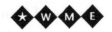

115 g/4 oz rice and millet flakes mixed
60 g/2 oz dairy-free margarine
60 g/2 oz unrefined light brown molasses sugar or honey
2–3 drops of vanilla essence
quantity of raisins, pumpkin seeds, dried banana chips,
    pineapple, mango, apricots (to choice)
toasted sesame seeds and pine nuts

Spread flakes on a tray and very lightly toast until just starting
to look golden. Remove from heat. Melt the margarine very
gently so as not to brown. Stir in sugar or honey, add drops
of vanilla essence and remove from heat.

Add the flakes and mix until they are well coated. Spread on
a baking sheet lined with baking parchment and bake in a medium
oven until they are golden brown and crisp. Leave to cool.

Add fruit and seeds of choice and mix. Store in a fridge
for up to 10 days.

Fruit and smoothie muesli

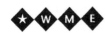

Serves 2

2 bananas, peeled and halved, *or* equal amount of pineapple,
    or raspberries, *or* a mix of white grapes and kiwi fruit
2 tsp white grape juice
large tub plain soya yoghurt
2–3 tbsp wheat-free muesli
few raisins (if allowed) or a piece of whole fruit, or carob
    bar (wheat-and-dairy-free)

Put fruit, juice and yoghurt into a processor and blend until
smooth.

Stir in the muesli. Top with choice of fruit, raisins or grated
carob bar.

Packed lunches and snacks

Savoury scones

Makes 5 scones

225 g/8 oz flour mix and 2 tsp wheat-free baking powder
  (see page 214)
pinch salt
60 g/2 oz dairy-free margarine
2 tbsp chopped ham
1 tbsp chopped sundried tomato (dried of any oil)
2 tsp basil leaves, torn
½ tsp wheat-free Dijon mustard
3–4 tbsp soya milk
1 egg, beaten

Sift the flour and baking powder into a bowl and add the
salt. Rub in the margarine to a breadcrumb consistency, then
stir in the ham, tomatoes and basil. Thoroughly mix the
mustard into the milk. Add the egg to the mixture and sufficient milk to make a fairly stiff but not too sticky dough.
Roll out and cut into 5 buns. Brush the tops with a little
extra milk and bake for 10–12 minutes (do not over-bake)
at 200°C/400°F/Gas Mark 6.

As a variation, the ham, tomato and basil can be replaced
with chicken, chives and sweet pepper.

Savoury tarts

Makes 6 individual or 6 slices

wheat-free shortcrust pastry using 170 g/6 oz flour mix (see
  page 220)
450 ml/¾ pint white sauce (see page 192)

Choice of filling:

(a) prawn, parsley and chopped cucumber
(b) flaked tuna and broccoli
(c) chopped cooked chicken and mushroom
(d) cooked minced beef, tomato purée and a little ginger
(e) chopped ham, green pepper and pineapple

Line a greased flan dish with the pastry or use individual dishes. Stir the chosen filling into the white sauce and fill the pastry case. Bake at 200°C/400°F/Gas Mark 6 for approximately 20 minutes or until the pastry is browned.

Fruity wild rice salad

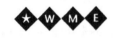

Serves 2

60 g/2 oz wild rice (raw weight), cooked
1 eating apple, chopped
1 tbsp herb dressing (see page 192)
1 large stick celery, sliced
30 g/1 oz dried apricots, chopped
½ mango, chopped
few sunflower seeds
few sprigs watercress

Put the rice into a bowl, stir in a little vinaigrette dressing over the chopped apple and add to the rice. Fork through, adding a little more dressing if necessary. Add the celery, mango, apricots and sunflower seeds and gently mix. Serve with a garnish of watercress.

Tuna and apple salad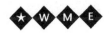

Serves 2

85 g/3 oz cooked brown rice
2 medium eating apples, e.g. Cox's Orange Pippins
2 tbsp herb dressing (see page 192)
200 g/7 oz tin of tuna (or required amount)
60 g/2 oz bunch watercress
washed few pine nuts

Core and slice the apples and dip in the vinaigrette dressing. Mix 2 tablespoons of vinaigrette dressing into the cooked rice. Divide between two plates and lay the watercress on top. Arrange portions of tuna and apple on the watercress and sprinkle the pine nuts on top.

As quick as you can

Serves 2

4 slices wheat-free bread (see page 214)
1 tin sardines (medium)
heaped tbsp cucumber, peeled and chopped
heaped tbsp chopped sweet peppers
1 tub soya yoghurt
watercress to garnish (optional)
salt and pepper

Flake the sardines, add the cucumber, peppers, salt and pepper and stir in the yoghurt.

Toast the bread slices, spread the sardine mixture over top and garnish with a sprig or two of watercress in the centre of each slice.

Apricot and pineapple snacks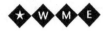

Serves 2

115 g/4 oz dried apricots
115 g/4 oz dried pineapple
115 g/4 oz desiccated coconut
1–2 tbsp white grape juice/apple juice
few drops pure almond essence (if not allowed, vanilla) little
desiccated ground coconut
Put the apricots and pineapple in a bowl, cover with boiling
water, leave to stand for 20 minutes, then drain.

Put the fruit and coconut in a blender, process lightly and
transfer to the bowl. Add the grape juice and almond essence
and mix together. Add more juice or coconut as necessary.

Shape into balls, roll in ground coconut and place in cake
papers. Place in the refrigerator to set.

Carrot, parsnip and thyme soup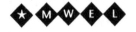

Serves 6

1 tbsp olive oil
280 g/10 oz carrots, peeled and sliced
280 g/10 oz parsnips, peeled and sliced
2 tbsp fresh thyme, chopped
2 tbsp fresh chives, chopped
1 clove garlic, crushed
½ bay leaf
1150 ml/2 pint chicken stock (see page 190)
salt and freshly ground black pepper

Heat the oil in a pan, and add the carrot, parsnip, thyme,
chives, garlic and bay leaf. Season to taste.

Cover and cook gently for 5 minutes, stirring occasionally
to prevent sticking.

Add the stock and simmer for about 15 minutes.

Transfer to a food processor and purée. Reheat, without boiling, when required.

A small spoon of soya yoghurt can be swirled into the soup before serving.

Sweet potato patties
Serves 3–4

450 g/1 lb sweet potatoes
1 egg
1 tbsp gram flour
¼ tsp salt
good pinch of nutmeg
oil for frying

Peel the potatoes and chop fairly small. Transfer to a blender and process until smooth. Add the egg, flour and seasoning and blend for 1 minute.

Pour a small amount of oil into the base of a frying pan and bring to a moderate heat. Drop 1 tbsp of potato mixture into the pan and fry gently for about 8 minutes or until golden brown, turning once. Drain on kitchen paper and keep warm while cooking the remaining mixture in the same way.

Vegetarian dishes

Harvest vegetable pie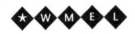

Serves 6

2 medium carrots, cubed
1 large parsnip, cut into pieces
115 g/4 oz small cauliflower florets
115 g/4 oz small broccoli florets
115 g/4 oz fine beans, cut into pieces
170 g/6 oz swede, cubed
85 g/3 oz cabbage, chopped
600–850 ml/1–1½ pints vegetable stock (see page 190)
1 sprig fresh thyme and 1 bay-leaf (or bouquet garni)
4 sweet potatoes
pinch nutmeg
arrowroot
salt and pepper

Place the carrots, parsnip, cauliflower, broccoli, beans, swede and cabbage in a large pan. Add the stock, thyme and bayleaf. Bring to the boil and reduce the heat to a simmer for approximately 15 minutes, or until vegetables are cooked.

Scrub the sweet potatoes, cook in a pan of slightly salted water and drain.

Discard the bay-leaf. Remove the vegetables with a slotted spoon and place in an ovenproof casserole dish.

Boil the stock to reduce by half and thicken with a little arrowroot. Pour over the vegetables to moisten, but not cover them.

Skin and mash the sweet potatoes, adding the nutmeg. Spread them over the vegetables. Bake at 180°C/350°F/Gas Mark 4 until the top is golden brown.

Stuffed peppers

Serves 4

4 good-sized peppers, red or green
2 tbsp sunflower oil
85 g/3 oz cooked rice, preferably brown
60 g/2 oz mushrooms, finely chopped
2 spikes chives, finely chopped
60 g/2 oz bean sprouts
85–115 g/3–4 oz water chestnuts, cut into small pieces
salt and pepper
olive oil

Heat the sunflower oil in a pan and add the chives and mushrooms. Cook for 3–4 minutes. Add the bean sprouts and water chestnuts and cook for a further 2 minutes. Remove the pan from the heat and transfer the contents into a bowl. Add the rice, season well and mix together.

Prepare the peppers, cutting off the tops to make lids, scoop out the seeds and core. Fill with the vegetable mixture and place the lids on top.

Brush all over with olive oil and bake at 180°C/350°F/Gas Mark 4 for about 20–25 minutes.

Peking mixed vegetables

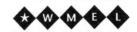

Serves 2

3 tbsp sunflower oil
1 clove garlic
25 mm/1 in fresh ginger, peeled and sliced
salt and pepper
1 large carrot, very thinly sliced
1 green pepper, de-seeded, cored and shredded
115 g/4 oz small cauliflower florets
60 g/2 oz prepared bean sprouts
60 g/2 oz water chestnuts, cut into small pieces

170 ml/6 fl oz vegetable stock (see page 190)
2 tsp Tamari (wheat-free soy sauce)
1 tsp brown sugar or honey

Heat the oil in a large pan or wok. When hot, add the garlic, ginger, salt and pepper. Cook for 1–2 minutes. Add the carrots, green pepper and cauliflower and stir fry for 3–4 minutes.

Add the bean sprouts and water chestnuts and fry for another 1–2 minutes. Stirring, add the stock Tamari and sugar. Check the seasoning. Cover and cook for 3–4 minutes.

Remove from the heat, turn onto a warm dish and serve with prepared cooked rice noodles.

Florence tart

Serves 2

4 or 5 slices aubergine
170 g/6 oz wheat-free shortcrust pastry (see page 220)
2 tbsp sunflower oil
2 garlic cloves, crushed
2 large tomatoes, skinned, de-seeded and chopped
1 medium courgette, chopped
2 tsp fresh chives, chopped
salt and pepper
2 tsp fresh basil leaves, torn

Lay the aubergine slices on a plate, sprinkle with salt and leave to sweat.

Line a 15 cm/6 in flan dish or individual dishes with prepared pastry and set aside to rest. Retain pastry trimmings.

Pour the oil into a pan and lightly fry the garlic for 2–3 minutes. Add the chives and courgettes. Rinse and pat dry the aubergines, chop into small pieces and add to the pan. Cook for 4–5 minutes. Add the chopped tomatoes and cook for a further 3–4 minutes. Season to taste, add the torn basil leaves, stir and spread the mixture over the pastry case.

Roll out the pastry trimmings and cut into strips. Place over the top of the tart to make a lattice effect. Bake for approximately 20 minutes at 200°C/400°F/Gas Mark 6, or until the pastry is cooked.

Vegetable kebabs with saffron rice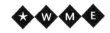

Serves 3

6 oz rice
2½ times quantity of chicken stock to quantity of rice (see page 190)
pinch of saffron
pinch of cinnamon
pinch of cardomon
black pepper to taste
1 tbsp sunflower oil
1 tsp rice vinegar
1 tsp fresh thyme
1 tsp fresh rosemary
salt and pepper

Kebabs:
175 g/6 oz courgettes
6 mushrooms – 2 per person
9 cherry tomatoes – 3 per person
1 green pepper, cut into 6 pieces, 2 pieces per person
1 orange or 1 yellow pepper, cut into 6 pieces, 2 pieces per person

Mix together the oil, rice vinegar and herbs. Stir well and set aside to allow the flavours to develop. If this can be done ahead of time, so much the better.

Put the stock, saffron, cardomon and cinnamon in a pan, bring to the boil and simmer for 3–4 minutes. Wash and drain the rice and add to the pan. Stir well and cook for the required amount of time. Drain, season with black pepper, put into a heated dish and keep warm.

Heat the grill to medium, arrange the vegetables on skewers and brush well with the herb-flavoured oil. Grill the kebabs, turning and basting frequently, until cooked and lightly browned (8–10 minutes). Remove from the skewers and serve on a bed of warm rice.

Mediterranean salad with penne

Serves 2–3

1 avocado, sliced
340 g/12 oz fresh tomatoes, sliced
340 g/12 oz green, yellow and orange peppers, thinly sliced
black olives
280–340 g/10–12 oz rice pasta (penne variety)

Dressing:
6 tbsp olive oil
3 tbsp rice vinegar
1 tsp wheat-free Dijon mustard
1 tsp demerara sugar
1 heaped tsp fresh marjoram or basil, finely chopped

Cook the penne in lightly salted water.

Place the ingredients for the dressing in a blender or shaker, mix well and chill.

Assemble the salad ingredients, drain the penne and fold into the salad. Pour over a little dressing and sprinkle well with herbs. Serve any remaining dressing separately or refrigerate for future use.

Pasta with lentil and courgette sauce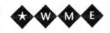
Serves 2–3

115 g/4 oz lentils
1 tbsp sunflower oil
1 clove garlic, crushed
10 cm/4 in piece of leek, sliced
1 dessertspoon fresh chives, chopped
280 g/10 oz courgettes, chopped
400 g/14 oz tin or jar plum tomatoes
good pinch oregano
salt and pepper
340 g/12 oz rice pasta (spaghetti variety)
parsley to garnish

Soak the lentils overnight in 600 ml/1 pint of water. Simmer gently in the soaking liquid until soft.

Fry the garlic, leek and chives in oil, add the seasonings and courgettes and sauté for 10 minutes. Then add the tomatoes and lentils and cook for a further 10–15 minutes.

Cook the pasta as directed, drain and pour into a serving dish. Pour over the sauce and sprinkle with parsley.

Chilli beans hotpot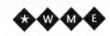
Serves 4

600 ml/1 pint vegetable stock (see page 190)
30–60 g/1–2 oz dairy-free margarine or sunflower oil
450 g/1 lb vegetables, e.g. swede, parsnips, carrots, celery and
    leeks, cut into small cubes
1 or 2 cloves garlic, depending on size, crushed
400 g/14 oz jar chopped tomatoes
2 heaped tbsp tomato purée
400 g/14 oz tin mixed beans (haricot, cannellini, kidney, etc.)
salt and pepper
chilli powder to taste

1 large sweet potato
parsley to garnish

Heat the oil in a pan and add the vegetables and garlic. Sweat for a few minutes but do not brown. Add the tomatoes, purée, seasoning and stock and stir. Add the beans and simmer over a low heat for 20–25 minutes.

Meanwhile, scrub the sweet potato well and steam or boil whole for 15–20 minutes. Drain and rinse in cold water. Slice very thinly.

Remove the beans from the heat, transfer to an ovenproof dish and adjust the seasoning as necessary.

Layer the slices of sweet potato over the beans, brush the top with oil and bake for 15–20 minutes at the top of the oven at 180°C/350°F/Gas Mark 4, or cook under the grill until browned.

Remove, sprinkle with parsley and serve.

Bean bourgignon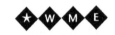

Serves 4

1 tbsp sunflower oil
1 carrot, sliced
1 clove garlic, crushed
3 spikes chives, finely chopped bouquet garni
½ tsp dried thyme
2 tbsp parsley, finely chopped salt and pepper
400 g/14 oz tin red kidney beans, drained*
400 g/14 oz tin haricot beans, drained*
450 ml/¾ pint vegetable stock (see page 190)
300 ml/½ pint red wine (if not allowed, increase stock)
1 tbsp tomato purée (increase to 2 tbsp if not using red wine)
1 heaped tsp soft brown sugar
60 g/2 oz dairy-free margarine
450 g/1 lb button mushrooms
½ tsp dried oregano

In a large flame-proof casserole dish, heat the oil, add the carrot, garlic and chives and fry for 6–8 minutes, stirring occasionally. Stir in the bouquet garni, thyme, parsley and season to taste.

Add both the beans, stock, wine, tomato purée and sugar. Bring to the boil, then reduce to a very low heat and simmer, covered, for 40–45 minutes.

Before the end of the cooking time, heat the margarine in a frying pan. When it is melted, add the mushrooms and oregano and fry for about 3 minutes. Using a slotted spoon, transfer the mushrooms to the casserole. Serve with boiled rice.

* Cooked fresh kidney and haricot beans can be used instead if preferred.

Asparagus stuffed pancakes

Makes 4 or 5 pancakes using a 15–18 cm/6–7 in heavy-based pan

asparagus, fresh, frozen or canned, 3 spears per pancake
85 g/ 3 oz flour mix (see page 212)
pinch salt
1 egg
3–4 tbsp soya milk
1 tbsp sunflower oil (preferably 'buttery' variety) for cooking
2 tbsp soya cream
½ tsp wheat-free Dijon mustard

Steam the asparagus until it is just tender and keep warm.

Sift the flour into a bowl, add the salt and make a centre well. Add the egg and a little milk and beat with a metal spoon until smooth. Add a little more milk until a creamy consistency is reached, then add the sunflower oil. The consistency should now be a thin cream. Place in the refrigerator to rest and chill.

Brush a pan with oil and heat to a very high temperature. Beat the batter and pour in the right amount for the size of the pan. Place the pan over the heat and cook the batter, turning. When the edges are brown lift the pancake and cook the underside. When both sides are cooked, remove and keep warm.

Cook the remaining batter in the same way. Stack the pancakes with leaves of baking parchment in between to prevent them sticking together.

Stir the mustard into the cream. Place a pancake on a warmed plate and lay asparagus spears in the centre. Pour 2 tsp of the cream mixture over the asparagus and fold the pancake over. Repeat with the remaining pancakes.

Mushroom fritters

Serves 2

115 g/4 oz mushrooms, wiped clean and finely chopped
60 g/2 oz wheat-free flour mix (see page 212)
½ tsp wheat-free baking powder (see page 214)
good pinch salt
1 egg
1 dessertspoon sunflower oil (preferably 'buttery' variety)
1 dessertspoon soya milk
little extra oil for frying

Mix together the flour, baking powder and salt. Stir in the chopped mushrooms.

Mix the egg with the milk, make a well in the flour mix and add the egg and milk mixture. Beat well together, add the oil and mix well.

Heat some oil in a heavy-bottomed pan. Fry a spoonful of the mixture until cooked and lightly browned, turning once. Drain on kitchen paper and serve immediately.

These fritters make a good accompaniment to a main course salad.

Butter bean curry

Serves 4

225 g/8 oz butter beans
1 tsp cumin seeds
3 tbsp sunflower oil
1 onion, chopped
30 g/1 oz fresh ginger, chopped
2 cloves garlic, crushed
1 tsp ground cumin
1 chilli, chopped
1 tsp ground coriander
½ tsp turmeric
4 cloves
450 g/1 lb tomatoes, skinned and chopped
2 tsp garam masala
salt and pepper

Soak the beans overnight. Then drain, rinse and cook in plenty of fresh water until tender – about 20 minutes. Drain and cover.

Dry roast the cumin seeds in a heavy-bottomed pan until they darken. Set aside.

Heat the oil in a pan and fry the onions until soft. Add the ginger and garlic and cook for 2 minutes. Add the cumin, chilli, coriander, turmeric and cloves, the tomatoes and 300 ml/½ pint water and cook until the tomatoes are soft. Mix with the beans and cook for a further 15 minutes.

Just before serving, stir in the garam masala and season to taste. Serve with rice.

Note: If you prefer a milder curry, omit the chilli.

Continental lentil rissoles

Serves 4

225 g/8 oz Continental lentils
2 tbsp sunflower oil
1 stick celery, chopped
1 large clove garlic, crushed
1 small green pepper, cored, seeded and chopped
1 tsp turmeric
1 tsp ground coriander
1 tsp ground cumin
¼ tsp chilli powder
salt and pepper
rice flour for coating
extra sunflower oil for frying

Soak the lentils overnight. Drain, rinse and put in a large pan with 280 ml/½ pint of water. Bring to the boil, then simmer gently until the lentils are tender and have absorbed all the liquid – about 30–45 minutes.

Heat the oil in a pan and add the celery, garlic and green pepper. Cook for 5 minutes. Stir in the turmeric, coriander, cumin and chilli powder and cook for 2 minutes. Add the vegetable and spice mixture to the cooked lentils. Stir well and season to taste. Leave to cool.

Mould the mixture into small rissoles and coat evenly with flour. Heat some oil in a frying pan. Fry the rissoles until they are well browned and cooked through. Drain on absorbent paper before serving with brown rice and a crisp salad.

The rissoles can also be served cold.

Tagliatelle with watercress sauce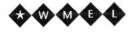

Serves 4

280 g/10 oz tagliatelle, wheat, corn and dairy free
1 clove garlic
6 anchovies soaked in water and well rinsed
1 tsp capers drained and well rinsed
85–115 g/3–4 oz watercress
a little walnut oil, if allowed, or light olive oil
a few toasted pine nuts

Cook the tagliatelle following packet instructions. Put garlic, anchovies and capers into a food processor and process until well blended. Add the watercress and seasoning to taste. With the motor running, drizzle in a little oil to form a soft paste, and add 4 tbsp of the pasta cooking water. Check seasoning.

Drain the pasta, return to the pan, add the sauce and stir. Remove to a warm serving dish and sprinkle with pine nuts.

Main course salad

Serves 4–6

170 g/6 oz white cabbage, shredded
85 g/3 oz carrots, cut into thin julienne strips
1 green pepper, cut into small pieces
1 yellow pepper, cut into small pieces
2 sticks celery, washed and cut into small chunks
a few bean sprouts, washed
30 g/1 oz sultanas
30 g/1 oz dried ready-to-eat apricots
30 g/1 oz toasted sunflower seeds

Dressing:

1 small tub of soya yoghurt
1 tbsp gluten-free mustard with balsamic vinegar

1 tsp sweet rice vinegar
good pinch paprika pepper

Mix all the salad ingredients in a salad bowl.

Blend all the dressing ingredients together and refrigerate until ready to serve. Pour a little over the salad and serve the rest of the dressing separately in a sauce boat.

Tasty courgette fritters

Serves 4

450 g/1 lb courgettes, washed and trimmed
½ onion, chopped, or 6 spikes of chives, chopped
light olive oil
3 medium-sized stems of rosemary
a pinch of ground cumin
salt and pepper
2 eggs
30 g/1 oz arrowroot or potato flour (Farina)
1 tbsp gluten-free flour mix

Grate the courgettes over a large mixing bowl. Heat I tbsp of oil in a frying pan, add the onions and sauté for a few minutes until soft but do not allow to colour. If using chives, add to the pan and stir over a low heat for 1 minute to flavour the oil. Add contents of the pan to the courgettes and mix well.

Pull rosemary leaves from stems. Chop finely and add to mixture.

In a small bowl, blend the arrowroot or potato flour into 2 tbsp cold water, stir into courgettes. Mix in the egg yolks, seasoning, flour and 1 tbsp oil. Combine gently but well. Whisk the egg whites until stiff and fold into the courgettes. Heat approximately 4 tbsp oil in a pan. Add 1 tbsp batter for each fritter. Flatten slightly and fry for 2–3 minutes on each side, or until golden. Drain on kitchen paper.

Cauliflower salad

Serves 4–6

1 medium-sized cauliflower
3 tbsp sunflower oil
1½ tbsp sweet rice vinegar
1 tsp honey
iceberg lettuce
a little shredded white cabbage
a little grated carrot
watercress, washed and coarse stalks removed
2 tbsp fresh parsley, chopped
2 hard-boiled eggs
8–10 cherry tomatoes
salt and freshly ground black pepper
pinch cinnamon
Parmesan cheese (if allowed)

Wash the cauliflower and break into florets. Cook in salted water or steam until just tender. Drain well.

Mix the oil, vinegar, honey, pinch of cinnamon and seasoning and pour over warm cauliflower. Leave to cool.

Wash the lettuce, finely shred the white cabbage and mix with carrot, watercress and parsley.

Put into base of dish, pile cauliflower in the centre and garnish with tomatoes and sliced egg.

Sprinkle a little parsley over the cauliflower. To finish, grate some Parmesan cheese over the cauliflower (if allowed).

Bermuda brochettes

Serves 4–6

1 packet tofu, cut into small cubes
1 small pineapple, peeled and cut into cubes
1 medium mango, cut into cubes

115 g/4 oz seedless black grapes
115 g/4 oz mango chutney (Sharwoods chutney is wheat-free)

Thread skewers alternately with the tofu, pineapple, grapes and mango. Brush well with mango chutney. Grill for about 5 minutes until very hot and just brown. Serve on a bed of saffron rice strewn with freshly chopped herbs.

If liked, mix a small amount of white grape/pineapple juice with a dash of Balsamic vinegar and drizzle over finished dish.

Tofu casserole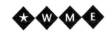

Serves 2–3

4 tbsp olive oil
1 packet tofu
425 g/15 oz can plum tomatoes
450 ml/¾ pint light vegetable stock
1 tbsp tomato purée
1 tsp sugar
2 level tsp dried oregano
115 g/4 oz fennel, cut into 1 cm/½ in dice
115 g/4 oz cauliflower cut into small florets
85 g/3 oz baby broad beans
60 g/2 oz celery, chopped
salt and pepper

Drain the tofu and cut into small cubes. In a non-stick pan, fry the tofu and celery in olive oil until tofu is browned and celery is softened.

Remove from pan, add tomatoes, stock, purée, herbs and sugar.

Deglace the pan by adding a very little water and scraping all the pieces on the bottom and sides of the pan into the juices, and bring contents to a gentle simmer. Add the vegetables, tofu and celery and continue to simmer for about 8 minutes or until the vegetables are just cooked.

Remove from the heat and serve on a bed of rice or stir in 60 g/2 oz of drained, freshly cooked wheat-free pasta.

Baked stuffed tomatoes

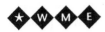

Serves 2

4 medium-sized firm tomatoes
2 heaped tbsp cooked brown rice
1 tbsp chopped green pepper
1 tbsp grated celeriac (if not available, finely chopped celery)
1 tbsp mushrooms, finely chopped
1 dessertspoon parsley
1 heaped tsp fresh thyme
salt and pepper
a small knob milk-free margarine
oil for brushing

Wash the tomatoes, cut off the tops for lids and scoop out the seeds.

Mix together the rice, pepper, celeriac, mushrooms and herbs. Season to taste. Pile the mixture into the tomato cases, put a knob of margarine on top of the filling and replace the lid.

Stand the tomatoes in a square or rectangular dish, brush lightly over each one with oil, and cover with lid or tin foil.

Put into a fairly hot oven and leave for 15 minutes. Remove lid or foil and continue baking for 8 minutes or until crisp but not wrinkled.

Serve with salad garnish for a starter or with full salad and crispy wheat-free bread for a supper dish.

Baked Italian salad

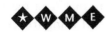

Serves 2

1 medium-sized aubergine
2 medium-sized courgettes

2 large tomatoes, sliced
fresh oregano and basil, chopped
olive oil
salt and pepper
toasted pine nuts

Prepare and slice the aubergines and courgettes, sprinkle with salt and leave to sweat.

When ready to bake, rinse and dry the vegetables, line an ovenproof dish with the aubergine slices, then line with the courgette slices followed by the tomato slices. Repeat, sprinkling the herbs and seasoning between each layer until all the slices have been used.

Drizzle a little olive oil over and bake for 20–25 minutes in a moderate oven or until the vegetables are cooked and tinged lightly brown.

Remove from the oven and sprinkle with pine nuts.

Vegetable salad with pasta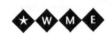

Serves 4

170 g/6 oz broccoli
dwarf beans
baby broad beans
115 g/4 oz mangetout
2 medium courgettes
8 oz wheat-free pasta, such as bavette or fusilli
Basil tomato sauce (see page 195)

Trim broccoli into bite-size pieces. Trim beans and cut into 4 cm/1½ in pieces. Trim mangetout and slice courgettes.

If using frozen baby broad beans, put into a pan of slightly salted boiling water, bring to the boil for 2 minutes. Drain, rinse in cold water, slip off the outer skin.

In an electric steamer, a tiered steamer or a Chinese steamer, steam broccoli for 5–6 minutes (but remaining crunchy), steam beans for 5–6 minutes, and mangetout and courgettes for 3 minutes, drain and refresh all vegetables in cold water, refrigerate.

Remove vegetables from fridge 25 minutes before serving, to come to room temperature. Gently warm the tomato and basil sauce by putting into a small basin and leaving to stand in a dish of hot water.

Cook pasta as packet instructions. Meanwhile, toss the vegetables in the sauce. Drain the pasta, transfer to a dish and pour over the vegetables and sauce.

Spaghetti with tomato and toffutti

Serves 3–4

280 g/10 oz spaghetti, wheat-, corn- and dairy-free
450 g/1 lb courgettes
2 tbsp sunflower oil
6 large ripe tomatoes, chopped
½ tub of toffutti with garlic and herbs*
1 tbsp sweet rice wine vinegar

(*Toffutti is made from soya and is a replacement for cheese. It is available in most health shops in plain, garlic and herb, and onion flavours.)

Cook spaghetti as packet instructions, but leave in cooking water.

Trim the courgettes and first cut lengthways and then into slices.

Heat the oil in a frying pan or wok and fry the courgettes for 3–4 minutes.

Add the tomatoes and 3–4 tbsp of pasta water to a sauce-like consistency. Cook for 3 minutes until the tomatoes begin to soften.

Remove from the heat and stir in the toffutti and vinegar. Season to taste.

Drain the spaghetti well and add to the mixture. Fold to combine and serve in warm bowls.

Budget recipes

Savoury crumble

Serves 2

340 g/12 oz minced meat
1 tbsp sunflower oil
1 large carrot, chopped
1 large/2 small sticks celery, chopped
1 dessertspoon wheat-free Worcester sauce
2 tbsp tomato purée
2 tsp fresh chives
pinch thyme
150 ml/¼ pint stock (see page 190)
salt and pepper
little arrowroot

Topping:
85 g/3 oz flour mix (see page 213 or use a mixture of rice,
  soya and gram flours)
40 g/1½ oz dairy-free margarine
30 g/1 oz wheat-free breadcrumbs (see page 214)
1 tsp mixed herbs
salt and pepper

Heat the oil in a pan, add the minced meat and cook until
sealed. Then add the carrots, celery, Worcester sauce, tomato
purée, chives, thyme and stock and simmer for 15–20 minutes.
Season to taste and thicken with a little arrowroot if necessary. Turn into an ovenproof dish.

Rub the margarine into the flour, add the breadcrumbs,
mixed herbs and seasoning. Spread this crumble mix over the
meat, smooth the top and bake for 45 minutes to an hour
on 180°C/350°F/Gas Mark 4.

Chicken livers with rice noodles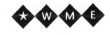

Serves 2

340 g/12 oz chicken livers, washed, prepared and cut into
   strips
115 g/4 oz unsmoked bacon pieces
2 tsp sunflower oil
60 g/2 oz mushrooms chopped
400 g/14 oz tin or jar chopped tomatoes
⅓ small green pepper, seeded, cored and chopped
2 tsp chopped dried herbs
30 g/1 oz gram flour
salt and pepper
rice noodles

Dust the chicken livers well with seasoned flour.

Heat the oil in a pan or wok and gently fry the bacon for
2–3 minutes. Remove to an ovenproof dish and add the green
pepper and mushrooms to the pan. Lightly fry for 2 minutes,
then add the liver, tomatoes and herbs. Cook for a further 2
minutes.

Season to taste and transfer to the dish with the bacon. Cover
and bake for 25–30 minutes at 180°C/350°F/Gas Mark 4.

Cook the noodles as directed and serve with the liver.

Mexican bean stew

Serves 2

225 g/8 oz minced beef
1 tbsp sunflower oil
115 g/4 oz red/green/yellow peppers, chopped
1 clove garlic, crushed
1 tsp dried chives
small tin red kidney beans
small tin haricot or butter beans
small tin chopped tomatoes

chilli powder to taste
225 g/8 fl oz stock (see page 190)

Heat the oil in a pan or wok. Fry the beef, garlic and peppers
for 5–6 minutes. Add the chives, beans, tomatoes and chilli
powder.

Bring to the boil, then simmer for 15–20 minutes. Serve
with rice.

All-in-one lamb hotpot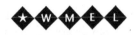

Serves 2

2 frozen lamb chops, thawed
little sunflower oil
1 large carrot, sliced
1 medium leek, sliced
a few frozen peas, thawed
115g (4 oz) cabbage chopped
1 clove garlic, very finely chopped
a sprig of rosemary
1 tbsp chopped parsley
450 ml/¾ pint stock (see page 190)
medium sweet potato, very finely sliced

Brown the lamb chops on both sides in a non-stick frying
pan, then remove from the heat. Mix together all the prepared
vegetables.

Place half the vegetable mixture in the bottom of an ovenproof dish, and put the chops on top. Lay the remaining
vegetables over the chops.

Stir the garlic, rosemary and parsley into the stock and
pour it into the pot. Cover with a layer of sweet potato and
brush with oil. Cover and bake at 180°C/350°F/Gas Mark 4
for 25–30 minutes. Remove the lid and continue cooking,
uncovered, for 30 minutes, or until the top is browned.

Pan-fried chicken livers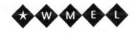

Serves 2

225 g/8 oz chicken livers
little gram flour for dusting
1 tbsp sunflower oil
½ tsp fresh chopped thyme
225 g/8 fl oz chicken stock (see page 190)
2 tbsp soya cream
1 tsp chives, chopped

Wash and prepare the chicken livers, pat them dry and dust
over with the gram flour. Heat the oil in a shallow pan, add
the liver and thyme and cook over moderate heat for 1 minute
to seal.

Remove the liver, add the stock and bring it to the boil.
Boil for 1 minute, scraping up the pieces from the pan. Reduce
the heat, return the liver to the pan and poach over a gentle
heat for 3–4 minutes, or until the liver is just cooked but a
little pink in the middle. Lift out the meat and place on a
warm plate. Add the cream to the stock and stir well.

Spoon the sauce over the liver and sprinkle with chives.
Serve with either rice or noodles.

Bacon and potato scramble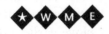

Serves 2

1 large sweet potato, scrubbed
a few small broad beans (fresh or frozen)
4 tbsp sunflower oil (preferably 'buttery' variety)
340 g/12 oz bacon pieces
2 small courgettes, thinly sliced
2 tomatoes, skinned, seeded and chopped into 25 mm/1 in pieces
1 tbsp chives, chopped
1 tbsp parsley, chopped
salt and pepper

Dressing: (omit for exclusion diet)
1 tbsp apple juice or rice vinegar
1 tsp honey
1 tsp wheat-free Dijon mustard

Cook the sweet potato in boiling salted water for about 8 minutes. Drain and cut into cubes. Boil the beans for approximately 6 minutes (they can be boiled with the sweet potato).

Heat the oil in a large size pan or wok, add the bacon pieces and chives and cook over a moderate heat for 3–4 minutes.

Remove the bacon from the pan, add the beans and courgettes and cook for 3–4 minutes. Add the sweet potato and tomatoes and continue cooking for 4–5 minutes, or until the vegetables are hot and cooked. Season to taste.

Return the bacon to the pan. Mix together all the ingredients for the dressing. Drizzle slowly over the scramble and sprinkle with parsley.

Baked porky pieces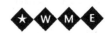

Serves 2

225–280 g/8–10 oz pork stir fry
1 tbsp sunflower oil
1 tbsp fresh chives, chopped
1 tsp fresh thyme
1 clove garlic, crushed (optional)
115 g/4 oz mushrooms, chopped
225 g/8 oz chopped fresh tomatoes or drained, tinned
    tomatoes and 1 tbsp juice
salt and pepper

Heat the oil in a shallow pan and add the chives, thyme and garlic (if using). Fry for about 2 minutes over a gentle heat.

Add the pork pieces and seal, turning once. Transfer to an ovenproof dish along with the mushrooms. Pour over the tomatoes and season well.

Cover and bake for 40–45 minutes at 180°C/350°F/Gas Mark 4, and then bake uncovered for a further 10 minutes. Serve on a bed of rice noodles.

Coley courgette casserole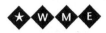

Serves 2

340 g/12 oz coley fillet, skinned
30 g/1 oz sunflower oil (preferably 'buttery' variety)
170 g/6 oz courgettes, thinly sliced
225 ml/8 fl oz fish stock (see page 190)
1½ tsp fresh mixed herbs (or ½ tsp dried herbs)
bouquet garni
1 tbsp arrowroot to thicken
2 tbsp frozen peas
2 large tomatoes, sliced
1 tsp paprika
salt and fresh ground black pepper

Cut the coley into 5 cm/2 in pieces. Heat the oil in a pan, add the courgettes and cook over a moderate heat for 2–3 minutes. Remove the courgettes from the pan and add the stock, herbs and bouquet garni. Bring to the boil and thicken with arrowroot.

Place the courgettes, fish, peas and tomato slices in an ovenproof dish, season with salt, pepper and paprika and pour over the thickened stock. Bake for 25–30 minutes at 180°C/350°F/Gas Mark 4, or until the fish is just cooked through.

Serve with rice noodles.

Spaghetti with vegetable sauce

Serves 2

rice spaghetti (enough for two)
approximately 450 g/1 lb vegetables (e.g. leeks, carrots, swede,
    parsnips, celery)
300 ml/½ pint vegetable stock (see page 190)
1 bay-leaf
3 or 4 peppercorns
pinch nutmeg
salt and pepper
chopped parsley (optional)

Prepare the vegetables and chop fairly small. Bring the stock
to the boil and add the vegetables, peppercorns, bay-leaf, salt
and pepper. Cook gently for 30–40 minutes, or until the
vegetables are soft. Add more water if necessary.

Remove from the heat and transfer to a blender. Process
until more or less smooth. Return to the pan. (A little arrowroot can be added to thicken the sauce if necessary.) Stir in
the nutmeg and leave to rest.

Cook the spaghetti for the required amount of time. During
the last few minutes reheat the sauce. Drain the spaghetti,
put on a warmed plate and pour over the vegetable sauce.
Sprinkle with parsley if using.

The sauce can be made the day before and stored in the
refrigerator.

Vegetable rice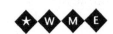

Serves 2

340 g/12 oz long-grain rice, cooked
60 g/2 oz sunflower oil (preferably 'buttery' variety)
1 orange or yellow pepper, seeded, cored and chopped
2 sticks celery, finely chopped
115 g/4 oz broccoli, chopped

2 large tomatoes, skinned, seeded and chopped
60–115 g/2–4 oz mushrooms, finely chopped
¼ tsp cayenne pepper
salt
1 tbsp fresh chives, finely chopped

Heat the oil in a large pan. Add the celery, pepper and broccoli. Stir fry for 8–10 minutes, or until the vegetables are
softened. Add the tomatoes and mushrooms. Continue
cooking for a further 5–6 minutes, stirring frequently.

Add salt to taste and the cayenne pepper. Stir in the rice
and combine all the ingredients. Continue stirring over the
heat for 8–10 minutes, or until thoroughly heated through.
Remove from the heat, stir in the chopped chives and serve.

Soups and starters

Gamekeeper's pot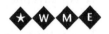
Serves 4

1 medium leek
1 large carrot
1 small celery stick
1 small parsnip
1 piece of swede
850 ml/1½ pints chicken stock (see page 190)
60 g/2 oz lean bacon pieces, finely chopped and soaked free
    of salt
1 tbsp cooked lentils
sprig of parsley
small piece bay-leaf
1 sage leaf
pinch dried thyme
salt and pepper

Wash and prepare the vegetables, chopping them into small
pieces.

Put them in a large saucepan with the bacon, lentils, herbs
and seasoning to taste.

Cover and simmer for 1 hour. Remove the bay-leaf, set
aside to cool, then liquidize to a coarse texture.

Cream of carrot soup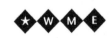
Serves 4

450 g/1 lb carrots, washed, peeled and chopped
1 stick celery, chopped
115 g/4 oz swede, chopped
60 g/2 oz lean unsmoked bacon, chopped
2 good spikes chives, chopped

850 ml/1½ pints chicken stock (see page 190)
30 g/1 oz dairy-free margarine
2 tbsp arrowroot
bouquet garni
salt and pepper
little soya cream or creamed coconut*
chopped parsley to garnish
* If creamed coconut is used, reduce the amount of salt added.

Lightly fry the vegetables for 3–4 minutes in the margarine; do not allow them to colour. Add chopped bacon and chives and continue to fry for another 2–3 minutes.

Add the stock, bouquet garni and seasoning and simmer for ¾–1 hour or until the vegetables are soft. Remove the bouquet garni and liquidize. Return to the pan and adjust seasoning if necessary.

Blend the arrowroot with a little water, add a little of the hot soup and mix well. Add to the contents in the pan and heat to thicken, stirring, for 2 minutes.

When ready to serve, reheat gently and swirl in the cream to the required consistency. Sprinkle with chopped parsley.

Asparagus soup

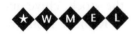

Serves 4

1 large bundle fresh or frozen asparagus
2 sticks celery
600 ml/1 pint chicken stock (see page 190)
parsley, chopped (to taste)
chives, finely chopped (to taste)
2 tbsp light olive oil or sunflower oil
salt and pepper

Chop the celery into small pieces. In a roomy pan, heat the olive oil, add the celery and chives and cook until the celery begins to soften.

Add the asparagus and stir round for 2 minutes. Pour in the stock to almost cover, add the parsley and season to taste.

Bring to the boil, then reduce the heat to a low simmer for about 30 minutes, or until the asparagus is soft.

Remove from the heat, leave to cool and then liquidize until smooth. When required, return to the pan and heat gently.

Mushroom soup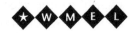

Serves 3

1 medium spike chives
400 g/14 oz mushrooms
300 ml/½ pint chicken or vegetable stock (see pages 190–191)
¼ tsp oregano
170 g/6 oz soya cream mixed with 115 g/4 oz cold water arrowroot to thicken
chopped parsley to garnish

Wash and slice the mushrooms. Put them in a saucepan with the stock, chive and oregano. Simmer for 20 minutes.

Remove from the heat and allow to cool a little. Add the soya cream and water mixture and stir well.

Liquidize the mushroom and stock mixture, return to the heat and thicken with a little arrowroot.

Add the cream mixture, pour into bowls and sprinkle with chopped parsley.

Cream of watercress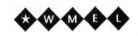

Serves 3

225 g/8 oz packet watercress
1 medium stick celery, finely chopped
1 dessertspoon sunflower oil
600 ml/1 pint chicken stock (see page 190)

1 dessertspoon arrowroot
salt and pepper
1 dessertspoon soya cream
chopped parsley to garnish

Wash the watercress well and check for tough stalks. Gently
heat the oil in a pan and sweat the watercress for 2 minutes.
Remove the watercress, put the celery in the pan and cook
until soft. Return the watercress to the pan, add the stock
and season to taste. Simmer gently for 8–10 minutes.

Mix the arrowroot with a little water, add 1 tbsp soup,
mix well and liquidize until smooth.

Return to the pan and reheat very gently, taking care not
to allow the soup to boil. When ready to serve, swirl in a
dessertspoon of soya cream and sprinkle with chopped parsley.

A sort of bouillabaisse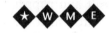

Serves 4

225–280 g/8–10 oz white fish fillet
600 ml/1 pint fish stock (see page 190) or water, or water
  and white wine (if allowed)
1 small to medium carrot
1 stick celery
8 cm/3 in leek
1 very small turnip
1 small tin tomatoes
1 heaped tsp tomato purée
1 small garlic clove, crushed
bouquet garni
sprig fresh dill, chopped
salt and pepper
parsley to garnish

Wash and skin the fish and remove any obvious bones. Wash
and finely chop all the vegetables.

Put the vegetables and garlic in a saucepan, lay the fish on top and add the stock, tomatoes, purée, herbs (except the parsley) and seasoning. Bring to the boil and simmer for 30 minutes. Remove the bouquet garni and check seasoning.

Serve in individual bowls; the fish will break into pieces naturally. Sprinkle well with parsley.

Chilled cucumber soup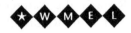

Serves 4

2 spikes chives, finely chopped
1 large cucumber, peeled and finely chopped
2 small to medium sprigs mint
750 ml/1¼ pint vegetable or chicken stock (see pages 190–191)
1 level tbsp arrowroot
salt and pepper
a little soya cream
green pure food colouring (optional)

Place the chives, cucumber, mint, stock and seasoning in a saucepan. Simmer gently for 25–30 minutes or until the cucumber is soft. Transfer to a liquidizer or blender and process until smooth.

Mix the arrowroot with a little cold water to a cream, add a little hot soup, mix well and return to the pan. Reheat gently, stirring, until the soup has thickened. Continue to cook, stirring, for a further 1–2 minutes.

Remove from the heat, allow to cool a little, stir in the soya cream and test the seasoning. If required, 1–2 drops of green pure food colouring can be added. Pour into a suitable sized bowl or tureen and chill.

For dinner parties, this soup can be served sprinkled with a mixture of finely diced cucumber, mint leaves and small green grape halves.

Lentil soup

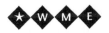

Serves 4

170 g/6 oz lentils
2 rashers streaky unsmoked bacon, finely chopped
2 spikes chives
1 small stick celery, chopped
1 small carrot, chopped
2 plum tomatoes, skinned and chopped
850–1150 ml/1½–2 pints chicken stock (see page 190)
bouquet garni
small knob dairy-free margarine
parsley to garnish

Put all the ingredients except the margarine and parsley in a pan. Bring to the boil and simmer for 1½–1¾ hours.

Remove the bouquet garni, transfer to a blender and liquidize. Return to the pan and reheat, briskly stirring in the margarine.

Serve sprinkled with plenty of fresh chopped parsley.

Cream of tomato soup

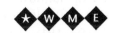

Serves 4

675 g/1½ lb tomatoes, washed, quartered and seeds removed
1 tbsp sunflower oil
1 small stick celery, chopped
1 carrot chopped
30–60 g/1–2 oz lean unsmoked bacon
2 spikes chives, chopped
600 ml/1 pint chicken stock (see page 190)
2 tsp tomato purée
1½ tbsp arrowroot
bouquet garni
4–6 peppercorns, depending on taste
1 tsp demerara sugar

salt
little soya cream
chopped basil leaves to garnish

Lightly fry the celery, carrot, bacon and chives in the oil for 3–4 minutes or until soft but not coloured. Add the tomatoes, stock, purée, bouquet garni and peppercorns. Cover and simmer for 25–30 minutes or until the vegetables are soft. Remove the bouquet garni and liquidize. Return to the pan. Add the sugar and season to taste with salt.

Mix the arrowroot with a little water to a cream consistency, add a little hot soup, mix well and return to pan. Bring to boil and stir for 2 minutes. Allow to cool slightly, then swirl in the amount of cream required and sprinkle generously with fresh torn basil leaves.

Cream of cauliflower soup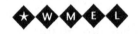

Serves 4

1 fresh white cauliflower
1 tbsp sunflower oil
600–750 ml/1–1¼ pints chicken or vegetable stock (see pages 190–191)
1–2 level tbsp arrowroot
salt and pepper
good pinch grated nutmeg
little soya cream
chopped parsley to garnish

Break up the cauliflower into sprigs, discard the green leaves and wash well in salted water.

Heat the oil and stock in a pan. Mix the arrowroot with a little water, add a little hot stock, mix well and return to the pan. Season to taste. The mixture should have a creamy consistency. Add the cauliflower and grated nutmeg.

Cover and simmer for 20–35 minutes or until the cauliflower is well cooked. Liquidize soup and reheat gently. Swirl in the cream and sprinkle with chopped parsley.

Harvest vegetable soup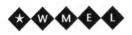

Serves 2–3

450 g/1 lb root vegetables (e.g. carrots, swede, turnip, leeks, parsnips, celery, celeriac, sweet potato)
stock, preferably beef (if not, chicken or vegetable – see pages 190–191)
6 peppercorns
good pinch grated nutmeg
1 bay-leaf
bouquet garni

Cut the vegetables into smallish pieces and put in a roomy pan. Almost cover with stock, then add the peppercorns, bay-leaf, nutmeg and bouquet garni.

Bring to the boil, skim off any scum then lower the heat to a simmer. Simmer for ¾ hour. Check that the vegetables are soft, remove the peppercorns and bay-leaf and leave to cool.

When cool, blend the soup to a coarse consistency. Adjust the seasoning and add a further pinch of nutmeg if needed.

Reheat when needed. This soup keeps well in the refrigerator for 2–3 days. It also freezes well.

Mushrooms in garlic sauce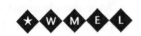

Serves 2

340 g/12 oz mushrooms, cut into chunks
2 or 3 cloves garlic (depending on size), crushed
225–280 g/8–10 fl oz chicken stock (see page 190)
2 tbsp sunflower oil (preferably 'buttery' variety)

⅓ tsp dried oregano
salt and pepper
little arrowroot

Put the oil in a medium-sized pan and heat. Add the mushrooms and garlic and sauté for 3–4 minutes over a medium
to high heat.

Add 225 g/8 oz stock and the oregano, reduce the heat
and simmer for about 8–10 minutes or until the mushrooms
are cooked. Add the extra stock if necessary. Season to taste.

Remove from the heat. Add a little arrowroot to some cold
water and mix with a little stock. Stir into the sauce to thicken
to a creamy consistency.

Serve with rice cakes.

Tropical ham salad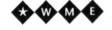

Serves 1

1 small piece each mango and pineapple, chopped
60 g/2 oz lean ham, chopped
lettuce leaves
salt and black pepper
few drops pineapple juice
toasted pine nuts or toasted sunflower seeds to garnish

Wash and dry the lettuce leaves. Season the pineapple juice
with a few grains of salt and some pepper. Lightly sprinkle
this over lettuce leaves and line a dish with them.

Mix the chopped fruit and ham together and place on the
lettuce. Sprinkle with pine nuts or sunflower seeds.

Potted ham

Serves 4

225 g/8 oz cooked ham, finely chopped
85 g/3 oz sunflower oil
½ tsp wheat-free Dijon mustard
1 tbsp chopped parsley
salt and pepper
little dairy-free margarine, melted

Put the first four ingredients in a blender and process until smooth. Season to taste.

Remove and put in a suitable clean dish. Cover with melted margarine and refrigerate.

This mixture can be put in individual pots and used as a starter. It is also very good for packed lunches.

Weekday tuna pâté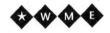

Serves 2

200 g/7 oz tin tuna in spring water
2 heaped tsp tomato purée
small knob dairy-free margarine
1–2 drops pure basil oil or 1 tbsp fresh basil leaves, chopped

Drain the tuna well and put it in a blender. Add the other ingredients and blend until well mixed and smooth. Put in a suitable ceramic dish, cover with cling film and chill well.

It is not necessary to use additional margarine when spreading this pâté.

Sunday salmon pâté

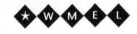

Serves 2

1 salmon fillet
6 peppercorns
good sprig parsley
good sprig dill, finely chopped
little fish stock (see page 190)
knob dairy-free margarine
3–4 drops rice vinegar

Place the salmon in an ovenproof dish, add the peppercorns and parsley and pour over a little fish stock. Cover with a lid or foil and poach in the oven at 180°C/350°F/Gas Mark 4 until just cooked through.

Remove from the oven and leave to cool in poaching liquid. When cold, remove the skin from the salmon and place the salmon in a blender with the chopped dill, margarine and rice vinegar. Blend until well mixed. Transfer to a ceramic dish, cover with cling film and chill well.

Dinner party starter

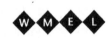

Serves 2

Sunday salmon pâté (see above)
small asparagus tips (4 per person)
few cucumber slices and mint leaves, to garnish

Vinaigrette dressing:
1 tsp wheat-free Dijon mustard
1 tbsp rice vinegar
¼ tsp salt and black pepper
½ tsp sugar
2 tbsp light olive oil

Put all the ingredients for the vinaigrette into a blender or screw-top jar, blend together and store in the refrigerator. Shake before use. (Any left-over vinaigrette can be kept in the refrigerator for up to 5 days.)

Line a small oblong tin or individual ramekin dishes with cling film. Two-thirds fill with salmon pâté and leave to chill.

Steam the asparagus for 3–4 minutes, keeping it slightly crunchy. Remove from the heat and drain. Turn out the pâté and place a slice on each plate (or turn out each ramekin onto a plate). Lightly dip each asparagus spear in the vinaigrette. Arrange 4 on each plate in a lattice pattern around the fish.

Decorate the salmon with cucumber slices and mint leaves.

Baked stuffed tomatoes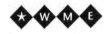

Serves 2

4 firm medium tomatoes
2 heaped tbsp brown rice, cooked
1 tbsp chopped green pepper
1 tbsp grated celeriac or finely chopped celery
1 tbsp mushrooms, finely chopped
1 dessertspoon parsley, chopped
1 heaped tsp fresh thyme
salt and pepper
small knob dairy-free margarine
oil for brushing

Wash the tomatoes, cut off the tops for lids and scoop out the seeds.

Mix together the rice, pepper, celeriac, mushrooms and herbs. Season to taste. Pile the mixture into the tomato cases, put a tiny knob of margarine on top of the filling and put on the lid.

Stand the tomatoes in a square or rectangular dish, brush them lightly with oil and cover with a lid or tin foil.

Bake in a preheated oven at 200°C/400°F/Gas Mark 6 for 15 minutes. Then remove the lid or foil and continue baking for about 8 minutes, or until the tomatoes are crisp but not wrinkled.

Serve with a salad garnish. If served with a full salad and crispy bread, this makes an ideal supper dish.

Sautéed scallops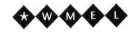

Serves 2

8–10 large scallops
a few drops rice vinegar
1 tbsp flour
salt and pepper
1 tbsp light olive oil mixed with 30 g/1 oz dairy-free margarine
watercress and cucumber to garnish

Trim the scallops (or get the fishmonger to do it for you when you buy them). Wash them well and dry them on kitchen paper.

Very lightly sprinkle the scallops with rice vinegar, season to taste, then toss them in gram flour.

Heat a large pan, add the oil and margarine and drop in the scallops; do not overcrowd them. Sauté until golden, turning once, for about 8–10 minutes. Transfer to a warmed dish and serve garnished with watercress leaves and cucumber slices.

Avocado with prawns in mango dressing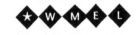

Serves 3–4

1 large mango
1–2 tbsp white grape juice
1 tbsp sunflower oil

salt and black pepper
225 g /8 oz large peeled prawns
2 small avocados, washed, peeled and sliced
watercress and lambs lettuce

Prepare the mango and cut into thin slices, setting aside two
slices for each serving. Put remainder into a processor, add
the grape juice and oil, season well and blend to a purée.
Remove to a dish and add the prawns. Fan slices of avocado
alternately with the mango on one side of each plate, and
place a small bed of watercress and lambs lettuce on the other
side. Spoon some of the prawns onto the leaves, and grind
over some black pepper.

Note: This is a good dinner party starter.

Fish

Baked trout with cucumber sauce

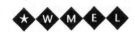

Serves 2

2 trout, cleaned
2 small bay-leaves
30 g/1 oz dairy-free margarine, melted
2 sprigs dill
salt and pepper
1 medium cucumber
little olive oil
little white grape juice or apple juice

Wash and dry the trout, removing the head and tail if wished. Sprinkle the inside of the trout with salt and pepper and place the bay-leaf and dill inside. Brush inside and out with melted margarine.

Wrap the fish in foil and bake at 180°C/350°F/Gas Mark 4 for approximately 20 minutes.

Meanwhile, peel the cucumber and cut it into small chunks. Heat the oil in a shallow pan, add the cucumber and sauté over a gentle heat until soft. Remove from the heat and take out 1 tbsp cucumber with a slotted spoon. Transfer the remaining cucumber to blender and process until smooth, adding 1–2 tbsp grape or apple juice to reach the required consistency.

Add a pinch of salt and the reserved cucumber, mix together and serve with the baked trout. May be served hot or cold.

Stuffed cod steaks with watercress sauce

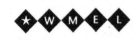

Serves 2

2 cod steaks
2 tsp multi-coloured peppercorns, crushed

1–2 tbsp olive oil
salt and pepper
170 g/6 oz watercress
small knob dairy-free margarine salt
pinch nutmeg
1–2 tbsp chicken stock (see page 190)

Heat the oil in a pan, wipe the cod steaks and brush with
oil. Press the crushed peppercorns onto both sides of the
steaks. (You can sprinkle the crushed peppercorns on and
gently roll a rolling pin over for the steaks to stick them on
firmly.) Season and place in the pan. Cook over a low heat
until the fish are cooked, turning once.

Meanwhile, remove the coarse stalks from the watercress and
wash well. Heat the margarine in a pan, add the watercress and
nutmeg, and sweat, stirring continuously, until wilted. Transfer
to a blender and process on the pulse switch to avoid over-
processing. Add chicken stock to reach the required consistency.

This dish is ideal served with baked sweet potato, carrot
and leek batons.

Tuna quickie

Serves 2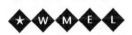

200 g/7 oz tin tuna in spring water
½–1 tsp wheat-free korma curry powder (check ingredients
carefully)
2 tsp olive oil
¼–½ tsp paprika
small tub soya yoghurt

Grease an ovenproof dish, drain the tuna and place in the
dish. Add the spices to the oil and mix well. Stir in the yoghurt.

Spread the mixture over the tuna, cover and bake for 15–20
minutes at 180°C/350°F/Gas Mark 4 until heated through.

Serve with saffron rice and steamed asparagus.

Plaice and celery parcels

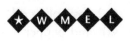

Serves 2

2 plaice double fillets, skinned
2 celery sticks, cut into thin matchsticks
1 carrot, cut into thin matchsticks
1 courgette, cut into thin matchsticks
115 g/4 oz chestnut mushrooms, wiped and thinly sliced
fresh parsley
celery salt and pepper to taste
2 tbsp vegetable or fish stock (see pages 190–191)

Heat the oven to 180°C/350°F/Gas Mark 4. Prepare 2 double sheets of buttered foil. Place the celery, carrot and courgette matchsticks in portions on the 2 pieces of foil and season lightly.

Put a portion of mushrooms on one half of each plaice fillet and roll it up. Place on top of the vegetables. Season the plaice and lay a sprig of parsley on top. Pour over 1 tbsp stock.

Wrap the foil over the fish to enclose completely.

Place in a baking dish and bake for about 20 minutes or until the fish is tender.

Seafood with noodles

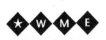

Serves 2

280 g/10 oz seafood salad or mixture of prawns, scallops and mussels
1–2 tbsp sunflower or olive oil
1 medium carrot, cut into batons
1 medium stick celery, cut into batons
½ green pepper, cut into fine strips
a few pieces fresh pineapple or mango
a good pinch ground ginger
a small amount of water chestnuts (if available)
1 tbsp fresh chopped coriander

1–2 tbsp apple juice
a good pinch paprika
4 oz rice noodles

Cook the rice noodles as required and keep warm.

Heat the oil in a pan, add the ginger and stir well. Add the carrot and celery batons and sauté for 5–6 minutes, add the courgette and pepper, then cook for a further 3–4 minutes. Add the seafood, pineapple or mango, water chestnuts if using, coriander and apple juice. Stir well and poach over gentle heat for 3–4 minutes.

Pour freshly boiled water through the rice noodles to reheat, drain and place on a warm serving plate. Spoon the seafood mixture over the noodles and sprinkle with paprika.

Seafood pasta salad

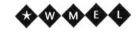

Serves 2

225–280 g/8–10 oz seafood salad
2 spikes chives, chopped
170 g/6 oz mushrooms, sliced
280–340 g/10–12 oz chopped tomatoes, tinned or bottled
1 dessertspoon sundried tomato paste
½ tsp powdered garlic
¼ tsp thyme, chopped
1 tsp basil leaves, torn into pieces
1 tbsp sunflower or olive oil
salt and pepper
4 oz rice pasta, cooked as required

Heat the oil in a pan and add the chives and mushrooms. Cook for 3–4 minutes over a moderate heat. Add the tomatoes, tomato paste, garlic, thyme and basil and season to taste.

Cook over a gentle heat for 6–8 minutes, add the seafood salad and poach in the tomato and mushroom sauce over a low heat for 3–4 minutes.

Pour boiling water through the pasta to reheat, shake well and transfer to serving dish. Pour the seafood and sauce over the pasta and sprinkle with parsley if desired. A bowl of green salad will complement this dish well.

Plaice turbans in mushroom sauce

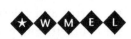

Serves 2

4 medium plaice fillets
salt and black pepper
350 g/12 oz mushrooms, thinly sliced
225 ml/8 fl oz fish or vegetable stock (see pages 190–191)
115–140 g/4–5 fl oz soya cream
pinch oregano
fresh parsley, chopped, to garnish

Wash and dry the plaice fillets, season lightly and roll up. Secure them with a cocktail stick if necessary. Transfer to suitable ovenproof dish.

Put the stock, mushrooms and oregano in a saucepan. Simmer for 6–8 minutes, until mushrooms are tender. Pour over the plaice, cover and bake at 180°C/350°F/Gas Mark 4 for 10–12 minutes, or until the fish is just cooked through. Remove from the oven, drain the liquid from the fish and transfer to a pan. Cover and keep warm.

Boil the liquid to reduce by about a third, then add the cream. Check the seasoning, stir well to mix and pour over the fish. Sprinkle generously with parsley.

Baked mackerel with gooseberry sauce

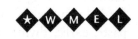

Serves 2

2 medium mackerel, cleaned and filleted

1 tsp rice vinegar
1 small knob dairy-free margarine
½ tsp dried mixed herbs
salt and pepper
225 g/8 oz gooseberries, topped and tailed
1–2 tbsp caster sugar
30 g/1 oz dairy-free margarine
115 ml/4 fl oz water

Wash and dry the mackerel fillets, place in an ovenproof dish and sprinkle the dried herbs on top. Season lightly, add a knob of margarine and pour over a little water and rice vinegar. Cover and bake at 180°C/350°F/Gas Mark 4 for 15–20 minutes, or until fish flakes are soft to the touch.

Meanwhile, wash the gooseberries, place them in a pan with the sugar and water and cook until the gooseberries have popped open and are beginning to blend (about 5 minutes). Remove from heat and beat in the margarine.

Pour a spoonful of the gooseberry sauce over the mackerel fillets. Serve the rest of the sauce in a sauce boat. Wild rice and a salsa of choice go well with this dish.

Salmon with roasted vegetables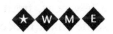

Serves 2

2 salmon fillets
4 medium vine tomatoes, cut in halves
115 g/4 ozs broccoli, in small florets
60 g/2 oz green beans, cut in half
1 clove garlic crushed (optional)
2 tbsp olive oil
1 tbsp rice vinegar
salt and pepper
a good pinch of paprika
grape juice or balsamic vinegar

Plunge the broccoli and beans in boiling water for 1–2 minutes. Drain and dry on kitchen paper. Heat the oil in a suitable oven dish. Place the tomatoes, broccoli and beans in the dish, sprinkle over the garlic and paprika, baste with some of the oil, and season to taste.

Cook for about 8 minutes at 200°C, basting again. Lay the salmon fillets skin side up on the vegetables, adding 2 tbsp of grape juice, balsamic vinegar, or water. Cook for a further 8 minutes until the salmon is just cooked through.

Serve sprinkled with chopped parsley and a sprig of dill.

Fish pie with sweet potato topping

Serves 4–6

450 g/1 lb sweet potatoes
450 g/1 lb floury white potatoes
tub of toffutti with garlic and herbs
150 ml/¼ pt vegetable stock (see page 190)
little cornflour or arrowroot
675 g/1½ lb boneless cod cut into large chunks
340 g/12 oz salmon fillet or 170 g/6 oz cooked peeled prawns
a few peas, fresh or frozen, cooked
some small broccoli florets, cooked
170 g/6 oz finely chopped celery, cooked
1 tbsp chopped parsley and dill
pinch of nutmeg

Cut the potatoes into even-sized chunks and cook for 18–20 minutes in lightly salted boiling water. Meanwhile, put the toffutti and stock into a small pan, and cook over a low heat until fairly hot. Add the blended cornflour and cook stirring constantly until thickened to sauce consistency.

Stir the fish, herbs and vegetables into the sauce and season to taste. Transfer the mixture to a suitable ovenproof dish. Drain the potatoes and mash. Season to taste.

Cover the fish mixture with the potato mixture and sprinkle over the nutmeg.

Bake at 150°C/300°F/Gas Mark 2 for 20–30 minutes, then place under the grill to lightly brown the top.

Salmon fillets with mustard cream

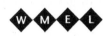

Serves 1

oil for brushing
1 salmon fillet per person
fresh parsley and dill, chopped
fresh fennel bulb, chopped
medium-sized potato
1 tsp sunflower oil
mustard with herbes du Provence (check the label that it is
    pure mustard seed and herbs with no added starch)

Brush a suitable dish with oil and sprinkle over the fresh herbs. Lay the salmon on top, skin side up, and leave to absorb the flavours.

Meanwhile, put the fennel into boiling water for 4 minutes. Remove from the cooking water, put in the potato and very lightly salt. When cooked, remove the potato and mash it, but reserve some of the cooking water.

Place the fennel around the salmon, add 2 tbsp of the cooking water per two pieces of salmon. Cover with foil and cook in the oven at 190°C/375°F/Gas Mark 5 for 12–15 minutes, depending on size of fillets. Remove from oven, place in a warm dish and cover with a lid or foil to keep warm.

Put mashed potato in a blender, add 1 tsp of sunflower oil, plus liquid from the dish the salmon was cooked in, and liquidize. Add mustard to taste, check seasoning and add hot water or cooking water from the potatoes to the required consistency. Reheat gently and pour over, or serve at the side of the salmon fillet.

Baked mackerel with tomato rice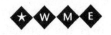

Serves 1–2

1 mackerel, prepared and in fillets
60 g/2 oz long grain rice
140 g/5 oz hot tomato juice
2 sundried tomatoes, finely chopped
85 g/3 ozs red and green peppers, finely chopped
a few frozen peas
a pinch chilli powder to taste

Preheat the oven to 180°C/350°F/Gas Mark 4.
    Place the pieces of mackerel fillet on tin foil. Season with salt and pepper, and add thin slices of lemon (if allowed).
    Fold into a parcel and bake in the middle of the oven for 10–15 minutes, or until cooked.
    Mix all the other ingredients together and simmer until the rice is just cooked.
    Place the mackerel and rice on a warmed plate and sprinkle with parsley.
    Serve with green salad.

Salmon and broccoli rice pie

Serves 2–3

Base:
170 g/6 oz rice, washed
½ tsp saffron (a small amount of other spices or herbs could be substituted)
1 egg, beaten

Filling:
225 g/8 oz tin of salmon
4 oz cooked broccoli
a few sliced mushrooms
1 egg, beaten

3 tbsp soya or rice milk
salt and pepper
chopped parsley

Put a pan of water on to boil, add the saffron and let it heat for 3–4 minutes. Stir well, add the rice and cook for the required time Drain well. Add the beaten egg with mix to combine. Press the mixture over the sides and base of a flan dish.

Drain the salmon and reserve the liquid. Arrange the salmon, broccoli and mushrooms over the base of the flan. Add 1 tbsp of the salmon liquid to the milk, add to the beaten egg and mix well, seasoning to taste. Pour into the flan, sprinkle parsley over the top and bake for 30–35 minutes in a moderate oven, or until filling is set.

Baked plaice with prawn and coconut sauce

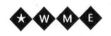

Serves 1

2 plaice fillets per person
85 g/3 oz prawns
30 g/1 oz milk-free margarine
115–150 ml/4–5 fl oz creamed coconut
1 tbsp mirren or sweet rice vinegar
1 level tsp tomato purée
2 tbsp fresh parsley, chopped

Wash and dry the plaice, and brush with some of the melted margarine. Fold the fillets in half and lay in an ovenproof dish, brush again with more melted margarine and season to taste. Bake in a moderate oven for 6–8 minutes or until cooked.

Put the creamed coconut in a small pan, add the mirren or rice vinegar, and the tomato purée and mix well. Heat gently and add the prawns. Pour over the plaice fillets and serve.

This dish goes well with new potatoes, broccoli and crunchy sugar snap peas.

Cod provençale
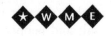

Serves 4

1 tbsp olive oil
4 spikes chives, chopped
1–2 cloves garlic, finely chopped
6 medium-sized tomatoes, skinned, seeded and chopped
4 fillets fresh cod, or any other firm white fish
2 tsp fresh basil, torn into pieces
2 tbsp chopped mixed peppers
1 tsp tomato purée
2 tbsp soya cream or suitable yoghurt
salt and pepper
1 tbsp fresh parsley, chopped
a few black olives (optional)

Heat the oil in a large pan and sauté the garlic and chives
for 2–3 minutes. Add the peppers and cook until peppers are
softening. Add the tomatoes, purée and a little water, or stock
if you have it (you will need a little more water if you are
using yoghurt rather than cream). Season to taste.

Lay the fish fillets on top of the mixture and simmer until
the fish is cooked (depending on size).

Transfer the fish to a warmed plate, swirl the cream or
yoghurt into the mixture, check seasoning and add olives (if
using). Pour over the fish and sprinkle with parsley.

Coated herrings with salsa
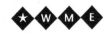

Serves 2

1 large herring, filleted
30 g/1 oz wheat- and corn-free porridge flakes
1 tbsp soya yoghurt
1 tsp Dijon mustard

Salsa:
2 medium tomatoes
1 piece of cucumber, cut into 1 cm/½ in cubes
½ green pepper
1 piece of fresh mango, cut into 1 cm/½ in cubes
2 tsp clear Mexican honey
2 tsp sweet rice vinegar
coriander to taste

Preheat oven to 190°C/375°F/Gas Mark 5.

To make the salsa, place the peppers, tomatoes, cucumber, mango and coriander in a food processor and chop until in small pieces and well mixed. Transfer to a dish. Mix the honey and vinegar and pour into the salsa. Gently fold into mixture to combine.

Cover and put in fridge to stay cool.

Put porridge flakes in grinder or processor and process to granule size. Mix the yoghurt and mustard together. Lightly season flakes. Dip the herrings into the mustard mixture and then into the flakes to coat. Place on a baking sheet and bake for about 15 minutes or until cooked. Serve with the salsa.

Tuna tomato cakes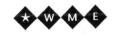

Serves 2

1 large tomato, skinned and chopped
115 g/4 oz tuna in spring water
115 g/4 oz cooked sweet potato
1 heaped tsp fresh parsley, chopped
salt and pepper
a little beaten egg (optional)
wheat- and corn-free flour for coating
sunflower oil

Mash the sweet potato with a small knob of vegetable margarine and a pinch of nutmeg.

Put the tomato, tuna, potato and parsley in a bowl, season to taste, and mix together until evenly blended.

Shape into 4 small cakes. (These can be made in advance and kept refrigerated until required.)

Dip in beaten egg, then flour or, omitting the egg, brush lightly with oil and coat well with flour.

Heat a little sunflower oil in a shallow pan and cook until golden.

Poultry

Chicken and apple bake

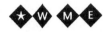

Serves 2

1 tbsp sunflower oil
340 g/12 oz chicken, cut into cubes
2 spikes chives, finely chopped
1 large stick celery, sliced
2 medium sweet potatoes
3 or 4 stems fresh thyme
1 medium cooking apple
1 small bay-leaf
30 g/1 oz Puy lentils
300 ml/½ pint chicken stock (see page 190)

Heat the oil in a medium frying pan, add the chicken and fry for 3–4 minutes, until lightly browned. Transfer to a casserole.

Put the celery in the pan, cook for 3–4 minutes, then add to the casserole. Peel, core and finely chop the apple, and add to the casserole with the chopped chives, thyme and bay-leaf. Add the lentils and stock. Stir well to mix. Cover and cook at 180°C/350°F/Gas Mark 4 for about an hour, or until the meat and lentils are cooked.

Remove from the oven and stir well for the cooked apple to thicken the sauce. (If it is not thick enough add a little arrowroot mixed in water and return to the oven until the sauce thickens.)

Steam the sweet potatoes until just tender, cool and rinse under cold water. Slice very thinly and layer over the dish. Brush with oil and put under a heated grill until the potatoes are lightly browned.

If preferred, the sweet potato topping can be omitted and the casserole served with boiled rice.

West country chicken

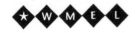

Serves 4

enough chicken drumsticks for 4 portions
300 ml/½ pint apple juice or white grape juice and 1 tsp
    caster sugar
medium sprig fresh rosemary
2 or 3 mint leaves
1 tbsp gram flour
1 tbsp light olive oil
salt and pepper
1 tbsp sweet red pepper, chopped
2 small courgettes, cut into rings
¼ tsp ground garlic
1 tbsp white wine (optional)
little oil for frying

Mix the apple or grape juice with the oil and season.

Place the drumsticks in a shallow glass or ceramic dish,
tuck the herbs around them and pour over the marinade.
Leave in the refrigerator overnight.

Remove the chicken from the marinade and drain. Toss in
gram flour. Heat a little oil in a pan, fry the chicken until
lightly golden and transfer to an ovenproof dish. Add the
peppers and courgettes. Stir the ground garlic into the marinade and white wine if using. Pour over the chicken and bake
at 180°C/350°F/Gas Mark 4 for 25–30 minutes.

Remove the chicken from the oven and keep warm. Boil
the liquid until reduced by one-third, check the seasoning and
thicken with a little arrowroot if desired.

Serve on a bed of rice noodles.

Chicken fricassée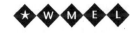

4 generous servings

4 good-sized chicken portions or required quantity of chicken
   stir-fry pieces
340 ml/12 fl oz chicken stock (see page 190)
½ sweet red pepper, chopped
few fine green beans, chopped
few broad beans, chopped
few asparagus spears, chopped
60 g/2 oz dairy-free margarine, melted
60 g/2 oz flour mix (see page 212) or arrowroot
170 ml/6 fl oz soya milk
3–4 tbsp soya cream
salt and pepper
chopped parsley to garnish

Wipe the chicken portions clean, place them in an ovenproof
dish, cover with stock and bake at 180°C/350°F/Gas Mark
4 for approximately ¾ hour, or until the chicken is tender
and cooked through. Remove from the oven, cool, then remove
the flesh from the bones.

Steam the chopped vegetables and keep warm.

In a saucepan, combine the margarine, flour, milk and
170 g/6 oz chicken stock. Whisk over a medium heat until
the sauce boils and thickens. Add the chicken, vegetables and
seasoning. Reheat and stir in the cream.

Sprinkle with parsley and serve with a bowl of rice. The
extra chicken stock can be saved, refrigerated and used next
day or put into an ice-cube tray, frozen and used later.

Curried chicken goujons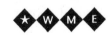

Serves 2

2 chicken breasts
2 or 3 medium spikes chives, very finely chopped

2 small cloves garlic, crushed
2 tsp wheat-free korma curry powder (check ingredients
    carefully)
½ tsp salt
good pinch cayenne pepper
1 heaped tbsp tomato purée
2 tbsp sunflower oil
gram flour to coat
parsley to garnish

Skin the chicken and remove any bones. Cut into thick finger lengths.

Stir the chives, garlic, curry powder, salt and cayenne pepper into the tomato purée. Brush this mixture all over the goujons, cover and chill for 1½–2 hours.

Heat the oil in a pan or wok. Coat the chicken on all sides with gram flour, place in pan and cook on a moderate heat for 6–8 minutes until lightly crisp. Serve garnished with chopped parsley.

Chicken in tarragon cream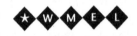

Serves 2

2 chicken breasts
1 tbsp chopped leek
1–2 tbsp sunflower oil
1 clove garlic, crushed
1 tbsp fresh tarragon
85 g/3 oz mushrooms, finely sliced
225–280 ml/8–10 fl oz chicken stock (see page 190)
115 g/4 fl oz soya cream
salt and pepper

Heat 1 tbsp oil in a pan or wok. Remove the skin and cut the chicken into cubes. Sauté in the pan for a few minutes until lightly browned. Remove and drain on kitchen paper.

Add a little more oil to the pan if necessary, and fry the leek and garlic until the leek is softened but not browned. Add the mushroom slices and cook for a further 3–4 minutes.

Return the chicken to the pan with the stock and tarragon and poach gently until the chicken is tender. Remove from the heat, season to taste and stir in the cream. Return to the heat for 1–2 minutes, until thoroughly reheated.

Serve with rice or noodles.

Chicken risotto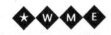

Serves 2

225–280 g/8–10 oz chicken, cooked and chopped
1 tbsp sunflower oil
60 g/2 oz bacon pieces, chopped
1 small leek, chopped
1 stick celery, chopped
1 green pepper, de-seeded and chopped
85 g/3 oz red kidney beans, cooked
60 g/2 oz mushrooms, sliced
1 clove garlic, crushed
225 g/8 oz patna or basmati rice
450–600 ml/¾–1 pint chicken stock (see page 190)
1 tbsp mixed fresh herbs, e.g. marjoram, basil, thyme

Heat the oil in a large pan, add the bacon and leeks and cook for 3–4 minutes. Add the other vegetables and cook for 2–3 minutes. Add the rice and stir until the rice is transparent.

Add just under half of the stock, and the garlic, herbs and seasoning. Cook over a moderate heat, stirring frequently. Continue to cook adding stock as necessary, until the rice is just cooked.

Add the chicken, stir well and cook until the liquid is absorbed.

Brittany chicken

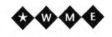

Serves 2

1 whole chicken breast
sunflower oil
1 tsp caraway seeds
300–450 ml/½–¾ pint apple juice
1 sage leaf
2 courgettes, diagonally sliced
2 medium Cox's apples, cored but not peeled
little dairy-free margarine
toasted pine nuts (optional)

Open out the chicken breast and beat with a rolling pin until evenly flattened. Brush the inside surface with oil. Heat a frying pan, place the chicken breast in it and seal, turning until lightly golden.

Transfer to an ovenproof dish. Add sufficient apple juice to come half- to three-quarters of the way up the dish (the chicken does not need to be covered), and the sage leaf if using, and cook in the oven at 180°C/350°F/Gas Mark 4 for about ¾ hour. Twenty minutes before the end of the cooking time add the courgettes to the casserole.

Heat a clean frying pan and add a little sunflower oil and a knob of dairy-free margarine. Thickly slice the apples and add to the pan. Sauté until golden, turn and cook until other side is golden. Keep warm.

Remove the chicken from the casserole, cut into 2 cm/¾ in slices and lay on a plate. Remove the courgettes. Place on one side of the chicken, with the sautéed apple rings on the other. Toasted pine nuts can be sprinkled over if wished.

Chicken with grapes

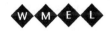

Serves 4

4 chicken suprêmes
1 tbsp flour mix (see page 212 or use sago, tapioca or gram
   flour)
1 tbsp fresh sage, chopped
150 ml/5 fl oz white grape juice
40–60 g/1½–2 oz dairy-free margarine
¼ tsp vanilla essence
salt and pepper
handful seedless grapes
8 oz either rice pasta or rice noodles
small knob of dairy-free margarine
1 tbsp fresh basil leaves

Check the chicken to remove any skin or bones, wipe clean
and if necessary flatten to an even thickness.

Mix two-thirds of the sage with the flour and coat the
chicken pieces. Melt the margarine in a pan and add the
vanilla essence. Stir well. Add the chicken and cook over a
moderate heat until tender and lightly golden brown.

Remove from the pan and keep warm. Cook the pasta or
noodles, drain, rinse and drain. Stir in the margarine and basil.
Meanwhile, add the grape juice to the chicken pan and mix
with the remaining pan juices. Bring to the boil and reduce
by half. Add the grapes and continue cooking for 1–1½
minutes. Pour over the chicken and serve.

Serve with roasted fennel and asparagus.

Turkey fusilli

Serves 4

675 g/1½ lb boneless turkey breast, cut into chunks
2 tbsp either rice or gram flour or flour mix (see page 212)
2 tbsp olive oil

1 clove garlic, crushed
½ green pepper, ½ red pepper and ½ yellow or orange pepper,
   each cored, de-seeded and sliced
225 g/8 oz chestnut mushrooms
1 medium courgette, sliced
400 g/14 oz tin or jar of chopped tomatoes
1 tsp oregano, dried
3 spikes chives, finely chopped
salt and pepper to taste
parsley to garnish

Coat the turkey in flour, then fry in the oil in a large pan until browned all over. Remove from the pan with a slotted spoon and set aside.

Fry the garlic, peppers, mushrooms and courgette in the oil remaining in the pan for 3–4 minutes. Add the tomatoes, salt and pepper. Bring to the boil, lower the heat and return the turkey to pan. Simmer gently for 20 minutes, until turkey is cooked and tender.

Serve with rice pasta, well sprinkled with fresh parsley.

Crock-pot chicken casserole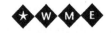

Serves 4

4 chicken joints
1 medium leek, finely chopped
1 dessertspoon sunflower oil
600–850 ml/1–1½ pint chicken stock (see page 190)
2 tbsp tomato purée
bouquet garni
salt and pepper
arrowroot to thicken

Remove any skin from the chicken joints and lay in a crock pot or greased casserole.

Heat the oil in a pan and cook the leek until almost soft,

remove with a slotted spoon and put in the casserole dish. Into same pan pour the stock, tomato purée and bouquet garni. Stir to combine the sediment from the leeks and bring to the boil. Thicken with arrowroot, season to taste and pour into the casserole.

Set the crock pot as directed or transfer to the oven and cook at 160°C/325°F/Gas Mark 3 for 1½–2 hours.

Chicken and sweet pepper casserole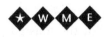

Serves 4–6

900 g/2 lb chicken thighs
2–3 tbsp sunflower oil
340 g/12 oz mixed coloured peppers, de-seeded and chopped
170 g/6 oz mushrooms sliced
1 stick celery, chopped
1 tbsp gram flour
2 tsp paprika
2 tsp tomato purée
450–600 ml/¾–1 pint chicken stock (see page 190)
salt and pepper
parsley to garnish

Heat the oil in a pan or wok and fry the chicken until lightly browned. Transfer to a casserole. Add the peppers, mushrooms and celery to the pan and cook for 2–3 minutes. Transfer to the casserole with a slotted spoon.

Add the flour and paprika to the pan, stir well and cook for 1–2 minutes. Add the stock, purée and seasoning, scrape up the sediment from the chicken and vegetables and bring to the boil.

Pour into the casserole, transfer to the oven and cook for about 1 hour on 180°C/350°F/Gas Mark 4.

Serve sprinkled with parsley. This casserole goes well with any kind of rice.

Pan-fried crumb chicken

Serves 1

1 chicken portion per person
1 oz wheat- and corn-free flour mix, seasoned
1 egg, beaten (or egg white alone can be used)
pure oat flakes, lightly toasted
a few pine nuts, toasted, optional

Put the toasted porridge flakes and pine nuts into a grinder and process to a fairly fine breadcrumb consistency.

Wipe the chicken portions, remove any skin and trim. Coat the chicken with seasoned flour, brush with egg and then coat in the crumb mixture.

Deep fry in olive or sunflower oil until cooked and golden brown.

Rosemary chicken

Serves 2

2 chicken breasts, on the bone
2 cloves garlic
a sprig of rosemary, approximately 10 cm/4 ins
chicken stock (see page 190)
2 large tomatoes, skinned, seeded and chopped
1 small courgette, cut into small chunks
1 dessertspoon olive oil
wheat- and corn-free flour to thicken, if required

Remove any skin from the chicken breasts and flatten to equal thickness. Heat the oil in a small frying pan and cook quickly, turning over to seal the chicken on both sides.

Preheat the oven to 180°C/350°F/Gas Mark 4.

Remove the chicken and place in a shallow ovenproof dish. Crush the garlic and add to the chicken. Wash the rosemary and add. Add sufficient stock to just cover the chicken, cover with lid and bake for 20–25 minutes, or until cooked.

Meanwhile put a little oil in a pan, add the tomatoes and courgettes and simmer very gently for 8–10 minutes, adding a little stock as required. Avoid overcooking or becoming too dry.

Remove the chicken from the oven, remove the rosemary and add the tomato/courgette mixture. Gently combine the liquid and thicken if necessary.

Serve with pasta and a side salad.

Balsamic chicken with summer salad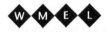

Serves 4

2 tbsp balsamic vinegar
4 boned and skinless chicken breasts
2 ripe peaches, stoned and sliced
a few green seedless grapes, halved
a mixture of baby spinach, lambs lettuce and watercress
torn basil leaves
olive oil
salt and pepper
small amount of fusilli pasta (wheat-, corn- and dairy-free)

Put 1 tbsp of the balsamic vinegar and 1 tbsp of olive oil in a dish and season well. Add the chicken fillets, coating them well in the dressing. Place the chicken fillets in a single layer, on a foil-lined grill rack and grill for 12–14 minutes. Turn over and grill for another 12 minutes or until the chicken is brown and glossy.

Spread the mixed spinach, lambs lettuce and watercress over a large platter. Slice the chicken and layer the slices over the green leaves. Repeat with the fusilli, peach slices, grapes and half the basil.

Mix the remaining vinegar and olive oil and season to taste. Add the remaining basil leaves, pour over the salad platter and serve.

Spanish chicken

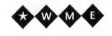

Serves 4

6 spikes of chives, chopped
1 clove garlic, crushed
1 tbsp olive oil
4 skinless portions of chicken
2 Cox's apples, cored and cut into chunks
60 g/2 oz ready-to-eat prunes
60 g/2 oz ready-to-eat apricots
150 ml/¼ pint of fresh pineapple juice
a few toasted pine nuts
chopped parsley

Heat the oil in a heavy pan, add the garlic and cook until soft but do not allow to colour. If using chives add them to the pan and cook, stirring, for 2–3 minutes.

Add the chicken portions to the pan and cook, turning until they begin to colour. Add the apples, prunes, apricots and pineapple juice. Simmer until tender (approximately 20 minutes). Add a little more juice or water, if necessary.

Serve sprinkled with chopped parsley and toasted pine nuts.

Chicken and carrot loaf

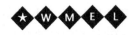

340 g/12 oz minced chicken
225 g/8 oz chopped parsley
4 medium-size carrots, chopped small
4–5 spikes fresh chives
140 g/5 oz cooked brown rice
salt and pepper to taste
300–340 g/11–12 oz soya yoghurt

Combine the chicken, half the parsley, 340 g/12 oz carrots, chives, rice and yogurt in a large bowl. Add seasoning to taste and mix to combine thoroughly. Press one-third of this mixture into the base of a suitable terrine dish. Sprinkle the remaining carrots over the top and press down very firmly with your hand. Add another third of the chicken mixture and press down firmly. Sprinkle the remaining parsley over the top. Top with the last of the chicken mixture and press down firmly.

Cover with foil and place the terrine in a larger dish. Fill this with water that reaches half-way up the sides of the terrine. Bake in a medium oven, for about 1 hour or until the loaf is golden brown. Leave to cool in the dish.

Gently ease round the sides with a spatula and turn the loaf onto a plate and chill. Can be served with salad for a packed lunch, or with steamed vegetables for a main meal.

Devilled chicken

Serves 2

2 chicken fillets
2 rashers low-salt, low-sugar bacon
115 g/4 oz chestnut mushrooms, wiped and sliced
Dijon mustard (wheat-free)
½ tsp clear honey
small sprig fresh thyme
a little chopped parsley

Preheat the oven to 160°C/325°F/Gas Mark 3.

Wipe the chicken fillets and beat until flattened and equal thickness all over. Brush one side with oil and turn over.

Mix a little oil with ½ tsp Dijon mustard and honey, to taste, and brush over the other side of the chicken.

Heat a heavy-based pan, add the bacon rashers and the thyme, and fry for 1 minute each side. Remove rashers from the pan, leaving the thyme in the pan. Add the sliced mushrooms and fry for 1–1½ minutes and remove.

Spread the rashers of bacon over the chicken on top of the mustard and honey dressing and fold fillet into three.

Bake in a covered dish for 20 to 25 minutes or until chicken is cooked through.

Serve with potatoes, and a mix of sliced green beans and courgettes.

Chicken and broccoli bake

Serves 4

4 chicken breasts, skinned and boned
1 egg white, lightly beaten
4 rashers lean bacon
1 tsp oregano, chopped
1 tbsp oil
10 fl oz chicken stock (see page 190)
115 g/4 oz creamed coconut
½ tsp wheat-free Dijon mustard
225 g/8 oz broccoli florets

Remove any skin and bone from the chicken. Beat with a rolling pin to flatten to even size. Brush the chicken with egg white, sprinkle with the oregano and wrap a rasher of bacon round each one in a spiral.

Heat a non-stick pan with a little oil, add the chicken and cook turning until brown both sides. Drop the broccoli florets into a pan of boiling salted water and cook for 3 minutes.

Place the broccoli florets in the base of an ovenproof dish with the chicken-in-bacon on top. Pour in ¼ of the chicken stock, cover and bake in medium oven for about 40 minutes, or until cooked.

Remove from the oven and keep warm. In a small saucepan, heat the remaining stock, add the creamed coconut and Dijon mustard, stir well and bring to the boil.

Remove the chicken and broccoli to serving plates, add the

juices from the oven dish to the saucepan, mix and heat thoroughly together.

Place a spoonful of sauce over the chicken and broccoli and serve any remaining sauce separately.

Chicken in leek and bacon sauce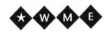

Serves 4

4 chicken breasts skinned and trimmed
4 rashers of lean bacon
2 large leeks, chopped
a small bay leaf
a few stalks of flat-leaf parsley, chopped
10 fl oz chicken stock (see page 190)

Place the chicken breasts in an ovenproof dish with a lid.

Cut the bacon into pieces and add to the chicken with the chopped leeks, bay leaf and half the parsley.

Cook in a moderate oven until the chicken is cooked. Remove the chicken and keep warm.

Place the bacon, leeks and stock in a blender and process to a smooth sauce. Re-heat and season to taste.

Pour over the chicken and sprinkle with parsley.

Note: A suitable gluten-, dairy- and yeast-free, low-salt stock cube can be used for this dish, if no stock is to hand. If required, the sauce from the blender can be thickened with flour or arrowroot.

Chilli turkey wedges
with pasta shells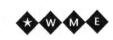

Serves 4

2 tbsp wheat- and corn-free flour
¼–½ tsp pure chilli powder, according to taste
4 turkey steaks

2 tbsp sunflower oil
1 clove garlic, chopped
1 tbsp tomato purée
2 medium-sized courgettes, cut into small chunks
450 g/1 lb cherry tomatoes, halved
600 ml/1 pint chicken stock (see page 190)
8 oz wheat- and corn-free pasta shells (gluten-free are readily
    available; look for SCHAR dairy-free shells)

Add seasoning and chilli powder to the flour. Cut the turkey
steaks into small wedge shapes and coat well in the flour. Save
the remaining flour. Heat 1 tbsp of the oil in a pan or wok,
add the chicken and fry for 7–8 minutes turning occasionally
until cooked and browned. Remove to a dish and keep warm.

Cook the pasta shells, as packet instructions, drain and
keep warm.

Add the remaining oil to a clean pan and add the courgettes and garlic. Sprinkle over the remaining seasoned flour
and stir in.

Cook for about 1–2 minutes, over a moderate heat, stirring.
Add the tomatoes and tomato purée, and continue cooking for
5–6 minutes, then add the stock gradually. Bring to the boil.
Return the turkey to the pan and simmer for 2–3 minutes.

Fold in the pasta shells and turn into a hot serving dish.

Chicken with sweet pepper and pumpkin crust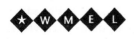

Serves 4

4 chicken breasts, skinned and boned
½ red pepper, seeded and finely chopped
½ yellow pepper, seeded and finely chopped
equal amount of pumpkin or butternut squash
1 clove garlic, crushed
large handful of fresh parsley, chopped
2 tbsp olive oil

a few toasted pine nuts or sunflower seeds
wheat-, corn-free tagliatelle

Wipe the chicken breast, and season. Place in a shallow ovenproof dish.

Combine the chopped peppers, pumpkin or butternut squash,
garlic and parsley in a bowl. Stir in the olive oil and season.

Spread to mixture over the chicken, spoon the stock around
the chicken in the dish and roast in a moderate oven for
35–40 minutes until the chicken is cooked.

Remove from the oven, sprinkle pine nuts over, and return
to the oven for 3–4 minutes.

Serve on a bed of tagliatelle.

Grilled chicken with fennel and mustard dressing

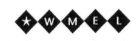

Serves 2

2 chicken breasts
1–2 tsp sunflower oil
1 dessertspoon mixed peppercorns
115 g/4 oz soya yoghurt
1 dessertspoon wheat- and corn-free Dijon mustard
115 g/4 oz fennel, finely chopped
1 tsp fresh dill, finely chopped
salt

Brush the chicken breasts with oil.

Crush the peppercorns and press them on to both sides of
the chicken breasts. Mix together the yoghurt, mustard, fennel
and dill, season with salt and refrigerate.

Heat the grill to high. Grill the chicken for 5–6 minutes
per side or until cooked.

Serve at once with fennel and mustard dressing.

This is good served with wild rice, mangetout and broccoli
florets.

Savoury lasagne

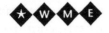

Serves 3–4

a quantity of wheat- and corn-free lasagne cooked, cooled
    and dried
a quantity of basil tomato sauce (see page 195)
340 g/12 oz minced turkey
2 tbsp sunflower oil
115 g/4 oz red and green peppers, chopped
2 medium courgettes, sliced and blanched for 2 minutes in
    salted water
soya yoghurt
1 tbsp fresh pizza herbs, chopped
½ stock cube, wheat-, dairy- and yeast-free
sesame oil garlic granules (optional)

Heat a little sunflower oil in a pan. Add the minced turkey
and cook for 3–4 minutes turning frequently to seal. Add
chopped peppers and tomato sauce, herbs and stock cube and
cook for 6–8 minutes. Check on the liquid and, if necessary,
add a little stock or water and stir frequently. The tomato
sauce must be sufficient to cover the lasagne well as some
can be absorbed during cooking.

Grease an oblong, shallow oven dish. Place half the turkey
mixture in dish and cover with the cooked lasagne.

Repeat with the remaining turkey mixture and more lasagne.
Spread a little yoghurt over the top of the lasagne. Lay the
sliced courgettes on top and brush them with the sesame oil.

Sprinkle with the garlic granules, if using.

Bake for 30–40 minutes at 190°C/375°F/Gas Mark 5 until
courgettes are golden brown.

Serve with green salad.

Beef

Braised steak with lentils

Serves 4

4 pieces lean braising steak
170 g/6 oz mushrooms, sliced
2 sticks celery, chopped
170 g/6 oz red lentils, prepared
600 ml/1 pint good beef stock (see page 190)
4 tomatoes, skinned, seeded and cut into pieces
bouquet garni
salt and pepper
1 clove garlic, crushed
little arrowroot to thicken (optional)

Spread a mixture of half the mushrooms, celery and lentils over the base of an oblong ovenproof dish. Lay pieces of braising steak on the vegetables and add the tomatoes. Sprinkle with salt and pepper and add the bouquet garni.

Add the remaining mushrooms, celery and lentils and the garlic. Pour over the stock, cover and cook at 180°C/350°F/ Gas Mark 4 for 2–2½ hours.

Thicken with a little arrowroot if desired.

Steak pie

Serves 4

450 g/1 lb lean braising steak, cubed
1 tbsp sunflower oil
1 large leek, finely chopped
225 g/8 oz mushrooms, sliced
600 ml/1 pint beef or vegetable stock (see pages 190–191)
1 tbsp tomato purée
bouquet garni

1 bay-leaf
salt and pepper
little arrowroot to thicken
wheat-free shortcrust pastry using 170 g/6 oz flour mix (see
    page 220)
little soya milk

Heat oil in a frying pan, add the steak and cook until lightly browned. Transfer to a casserole. Fry the leek and mushrooms for 3–4 minutes and transfer to the casserole. Add the stock, tomato purée, bouquet garni and bay-leaf to the pan. Stir to deglace and season to taste.

Thicken with a little arrowroot and bring to boil, stirring. Simmer until the gravy thickens, for 2–3 minutes, pour into the casserole and cook at 180°C/350°F/Gas Mark 4 for 1½–2 hours.

Remove from the oven and discard the bay-leaf. Place the steak and vegetables in the base of a 1.5 litre/2½ pint pie dish and spoon over 2–3 tablespoons of gravy, reserving the rest in a warm casserole.

Roll out the pastry and cut a 25 mm/1 in strip to go round the edge of the pie dish. Dampen the edge of the dish with water, place on the pastry strip and press down lightly. Dampen the top of the pastry strip with water. Place the rest of the pastry over the dish to form a lid and seal well round the edge. Cut two small slits on the lid, brush the top with soya milk and bake in a fairly hot oven until the pastry is cooked and golden.

Serve with the reserved gravy.

Goulash

Serves 4

450 g/1 lb lean stewing steak, cubed
1 tbsp oil
1 large leek, cut into rings

225 g/8 oz cabbage, shredded
2 tbsp tomato purée
170–225 ml/6–8 fl oz beef stock (see page 190)
2 tsp paprika
arrowroot to thicken
little soya cream
salt and pepper

Heat the oil in a medium-sized saucepan, add the steak and cook for 6–8 minutes to seal. Add the leek and cabbage and cook for a further 3–4 minutes.

Add the stock, purée and paprika and season to taste. Cover and simmer very gently for about an hour, or until meat is tender.

Remove from the heat and thicken with a little arrowroot to a creamy consistency. Stir in a little soya cream, check the seasoning and serve.

Rice noodles make an ideal accompaniment to this goulash.

Spaghetti bean bolognese

Serves 4

450 g/1 lb minced beef
115 g/4 oz bacon pieces, chopped
1 tbsp sunflower oil
1 stick celery, sliced
1 carrot, sliced
1 clove garlic, crushed
400g/14 oz tin or jar of chopped tomatoes
1 tbsp tomato purée
½ large tin mixed beans
1 tsp or cube wheat-free stock powder (check ingredients carefully)
2 tsp dried oregano
salt and pepper

Heat the oil in a saucepan and add the minced beef and bacon. Fry for 6 minutes, until beef is browned. Add the celery, carrot and garlic and cook for 3–4 minutes.

Add the remaining ingredients and simmer over a low heat for 30–40 minutes, then check the seasoning. Serve with spaghetti. This bean bolognese goes equally well with rice noodles.

Quickie beef patties

Serves 2

225 g/8 oz minced beef, cooked
3 spikes fresh chives, chopped
85 g/3 oz mushrooms, chopped fairly small
60 g/2 oz gram, or wheat-free flour mix
30 g/1 oz dairy-free margarine
1 egg, beaten
salt and pepper

Put the flour into a bowl and rub in the margarine.

Add the beef, chives, mushrooms, salt and pepper, and mix. Add the egg and mix well to combine.

Grease a baking sheet and put separate tablespoonfuls of the mixture on the sheet, without them touching. Bake in a moderately hot oven for 30–40 minutes until they are cooked through and crisp.

Serve with Vegetable Rice (page 112).

Beef cobbler

Serves 4

450 g/1 lb lean chuck steak, cubed
2 carrots, sliced
1 large leek, sliced
1 large stick celery, sliced
115 g/4 oz mushrooms, sliced

1 tbsp oil
15 fl oz stock (see page 190) plus 1 tbsp tomato purée
bay-leaf
salt and pepper
wheat-free flour or arrowroot, to thicken

Topping:
225 g/8 oz wheat-free flour
2 tsp wheat-free baking powder
pinch salt
60 g/2 oz dairy-free margarine
5 tbsp soya, rice or potato milk*
½ tsp wheat- and corn-free Dijon mustard

Heat the oil in a pan, add the steak and fry, turning occa-sionally, until brown. Transfer to a casserole. Add the vegeta-bles to the pan and cook for 6 minutes. Add to casserole.

Stir tomato purée into the stock, add the bay leaf and season. Pour over the vegetables and steak, cover, and cook in a moderate oven for 1 – 1½ hours. Remove from the oven and thicken with a little flour or arrowroot. Return to heat and, when thickened, remove and set aside.

To make the topping, sift the flour into a bowl, add the baking powder and salt. Rub the margarine into the flour until breadcrumb consistency. Mix the mustard with a little milk, then add the remaining milk. Mix into a soft but not sticky dough. Roll out and cut into rounds with a cutter.

Flour each scone well and place in a ring round edge of casserole.

Return to oven for about 10 minutes at 200°C/400°F/Gas Mark 6 or until scone topping is cooked and golden.
*If allowed, an egg can be used to bind the scone mixture but reduce the amount of milk, using same amount of mustard. Beat egg, milk and mustard mixture together.

Pot roast of beef

Serves 4–6

1 joint of very lean beef
2 carrots, sliced
2 leeks, cut into rings
2 sticks celery, chopped
170 g/6 oz swede, chopped
1 large tomato, skinned and chopped
340–400 ml/12–14 fl oz good quality stock (see page 190)
bouquet garni
1 tbsp sunflower oil
salt and pepper

Heat the oil in a large frying pan, add the beef and turn occasionally until brown on all sides. Remove to casserole.

Add the vegetables to the frying pan and cook until just beginning to colour. Transfer to the casserole. Add the tomato, stock and bouquet garni, and season well.

Transfer to a moderate oven and cook for 2–3 hours, depending on the size of joint of beef.

Remove the beef and keep warm. Thicken the liquid with a little wheat-free flour if desired.

Potted beef

Serves 2

225 g/8 oz lean minced steak (or good quality minced beef)
300 ml/½ pint beef stock (see page 190)
1 dessertspoon tomato purée
½ tsp grated horseradish
salt and pepper
60 g/2 oz melted vegetable margarine
30 ml/1 fl oz sunflower oil
a pinch fresh thyme

Put the sunflower oil in a pan, add the minced steak and sauté to seal. When lightly browned, add the stock, purée, horseradish and thyme and season to taste. Cover and cook over a moderate heat for 8 minutes.

Remove the beef from the liquid and place beef in a blender. Boil the liquid for 2–3 minutes to reduce slightly. Add a little liquid to blender and liquidize, adding a little more liquid until the required consistency. Put the beef mixture into a clean dish and pour over the melted margarine. Leave to cool and then refrigerate.

Note: This can be served in sandwiches, on individual shaped crackers, or in small pastry cases.

Speedy steak with zingy sauce and vegetables

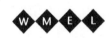

Serves 4

450 g/1 lb new potatoes, cut to equal size (if necessary)
280 g/10 oz broccoli, cut into small florets
225 g/8 oz carrots, sliced into rings
1 clove garlic, crushed
1 tbsp wheat- and corn-free wholegrain mustard
3 tbsp fresh pineapple juice
1 tbsp clear honey
4 thin flash-frying steaks
1 tbsp sunflower oil*

Boil the potatoes in lightly salted water and steam the broccoli and carrots on top, then drain.

In a clean pan, add the pineapple juice, garlic, mustard and honey. Mix together and bring to the boil, stirring until juices start to thicken. Add the vegetables. Remove from the heat after 2–3 minutes and keep warm.

Heat a griddle pan, brush the griddle and steaks with oil,

and season to taste. Cook the steaks each side for 1½ minutes. Place on a heated dish and serve with sauce and vegetables. *It is best to use sunflower oil as it is better suited to high temperatures.

Lamb

Lamb curry with pineapple and apricots

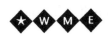

Serves 6

900 g/2 lb lean lamb, cubed
2 tbsp sunflower oil
170 g/6 oz leeks, cut into fine rings
2 tbsp gram flour
2 tbsp wheat-free korma curry powder (check ingredients carefully)
1 tsp ground ginger or 5 cm/2 in piece fresh ginger, grated
1 tsp ground coriander
12–14 fl oz chicken stock (see page 190)
225 g/8 oz creamed coconut
225 g/8 oz dried apricots
225 g/8 oz canned pineapple, drained
60 g/2 oz raisins

Heat the oil in a large pan, add the lamb and brown all over. Remove from the heat and keep warm. Add the leeks and cook until soft, without letting them brown.

Return the meat to the pan, sprinkle in the flour, ginger, curry powder and coriander and stir well. Add the stock and creamed coconut.

Bring to the boil, stir well and reduce to a simmer for 20 minutes. Add the apricots, pineapple and raisins, cover and simmer very gently for 1¼–1½ hours. Adjust seasoning and serve with rice.

Honey lamb

Serves 4

small to medium joint of lean lamb

Marinade:
170 ml/6 fl oz clear honey
2 small sprigs rosemary
170 ml/6 fl oz red grape juice
115–170 ml/4–6 fl oz concentrated pineapple juice
1 clove garlic, crushed

Mix together all the ingredients for the marinade. Place the lamb in a non-metallic bowl, pour over the marinade and leave in the refrigerator overnight.

Roast in the oven at 180°C/350°F/Gas Mark 4 for the required length of time (depending on weight of joint). Continue basting with the marinade during cooking.

Sweet and spicy lamb with rice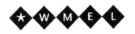

Serves 4

4 lamb steaks
1 tbsp sunflower oil
1 clove garlic, crushed
1 tin sliced peaches
1–2 tsp dried ginger (to taste)
2 tsp light brown or demerara sugar
pinch cumin
little arrowroot
8 oz white rice
1 tbsp fresh thyme, chopped

Heat the oil in a pan, season the steaks, and add to the pan. Fry for 3–4 minutes, turning once, to lightly brown both sides. Remove the lamb from the pan.

Put the garlic, cumin, ginger and sugar and half the peach juice from the tin into the pan. Heat through, add a little arrowroot to thicken and bring to the boil. Lower the heat to a simmer, return the steaks to the sauce and leave on a low heat for 10–12 minutes.

Meanwhile, cook rice as required, drain and stir in the chopped thyme.

Remove the steaks and sauce from the heat, stir in the sliced peaches and serve with a portion of rice. An ideal accompaniment is steamed or roast asparagus.

Irish stew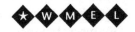

Serves 4

8 middle neck lamb chops or scrag end of neck lamb
900 g/2 lb sweet potatoes, peeled and sliced
450 g/1 lb carrots, cut into small chunks
450 g/1 lb celery, cut into small pieces
1 tbsp chopped chives
salt and pepper
pinch mixed dried herbs
vegetable or chicken stock (see pages 190–191)

Place half the lamb in the base of a casserole and add a sprinkling of chives. Then add half the carrot and celery followed by half the sweet potato. Repeat these layers, finishing with a layer of sweet potato.

Season the stock and pour into casserole to reach half-way up the side of the casserole. Sprinkle the herbs over the top.

Cover and cook at about 180°C/350°F/Gas Mark 4 for 2–3 hours.

Lamb kebabs

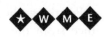

Serves 4

280 g/10 oz lean lamb, cubed
1 red pepper, de-seeded and cut into pieces
1 or 2 courgettes, cut into chunks
8 cherry tomatoes
8 button mushrooms

Marinade:
1 small tin vegetable juice
2 tsp wheat-free Worcester sauce (alternatively, use Mirrin –
    a sweet Japanese seasoning – or sweet rice vinegar, all
    available from good health-food shops)
salt and pepper
few fresh basil leaves, torn

Put the lamb in a non-metallic shallow dish. Mix the marinade ingredients together, pour over the lamb, cover and refrigerate overnight.

Remove the meat from the marinade. Blanch and drain the pepper and courgette pieces. Thread pieces of lamb, pepper, courgette, tomatoes and mushrooms alternately onto skewers.

Place the skewers across the grill pan, brush well with the marinade and grill for 20 minutes, turning and basting with the marinade.

Serve with saffron rice.

Lamb parcels

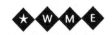

Serves 4

4 lamb chops, preferably lean and chump
4 large flat mushrooms
4 tomatoes, sliced
1 heaped tsp dried mixed herbs

1 tbsp sunflower oil plus a little extra for brushing
salt and pepper

In a pan or wok, heat the oil and cook the chops to seal
them until they are lightly browned.

Remove them from the pan. Lay tomato slices on squares
of foil, season and sprinkle with herbs. Lay a chop on each
base of tomatoes, top with large flat mushrooms and brush
with oil.

Fold the foil into parcels and bake at 180°C/350°F/Gas
Mark 4 for 30–40 minutes, or until the chops are cooked
and tender.

Welsh lamb-one-pot

Serves 4

4 lamb steaks, cut into chunks
340 g/12 oz leeks
340 g/12 oz broccoli
900 g/2 lb prepared new potatoes (cut in half if large)
2 tbsp wheat-free flour
1 tbsp oil
300 ml/½ pint apple juice
2 sprigs rosemary
salt and pepper

Season the flour well and then coat the lamb. Heat the oil
in a large flameproof casserole, add the lamb and brown on
both sides.

Add the leeks, broccoli and potatoes, pour in the apple
juice and add the rosemary. Bring to the boil and then reduce
heat to just simmering. Cover the pan and simmer for 35
minutes or until the potatoes and lamb are tender. Check the
liquid occasionally, adding a little more if necessary.

Lamb hash

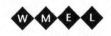

Serves 2–3

4 potatoes, coarsely grated
1 medium leek, chopped, or 2 tbsp chopped chives
2 tbsp olive oil
225 g/8 oz cooked lamb, cut into small cubes
30 g/1 oz pure dairy-free margarine
2 tsp dried sage
salt and pepper

Heat the oil in large frying pan, add the leeks or chives, add
the potatoes, sprinkle in the sage and season well. Cook,
stirring over a moderate heat until the potatoes are almost
cooked. Add the cubed lamb and mix well to combine. Press
the mixture flat and cook for 5 minutes without stirring. Dot
with the margarine and place under a hot grill until the top
is golden and crisp.

Serve, cut into wedges, with salad.

Curried lamb and rice fritters

Serves 2–3

280 g/10 oz cooked rice
280 g/10 oz small diced lamb
1 tsp wheat-free curry powder (or just a pinch, if preferred)
2 tbsp wheat-free flour
1 tbsp chives, chopped
1 egg, beaten
4 tbsp rice milk or soya milk
salt and pepper
sunflower oil

Mix the rice, lamb, spice, flour and chives. Add the egg and
milk, season well, and mix to combine.

Heat a little oil in a pan or large wok and drop spoonfuls of the mixture into the pan, flattening the rice so that it binds. Cook until crisp and golden underneath, turn and cook other side. Drain on absorbent kitchen paper.

This is excellent served with mango chutney (see recipe page 196).

Roasted lamb fillet with mint and apricot sauce

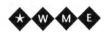

Serves 4

1 large lamb fillet, with fat removed
1 tbsp wheat- and corn-free wholegrain mustard
½ oz pure dairy-free margarine
150 ml/5 fl oz lamb or chicken stock
100 ml/3½ fl oz red grape juice mixed with 50 ml/2 fl oz of
   water
2 tsp mint jelly
1 tbsp honey
4 dried apricots, finely chopped
salt and ground black pepper

Blend the mustard with the margarine and spread over the lamb fillet. Place the joint on a rack in a roasting tin, adding 2 tbsp of water in the base of the tin. Roast in a moderate oven until cooked, for 20 minutes per ½ kg/1 lb, plus 20 minutes, or less if required pink.

Put the red grape juice and water, stock, mint jelly, honey and apricots in a small pan, and simmer until reduced by two-thirds.

When the meat is cooked, remove to a warm dish, pour the meat juices into the sauce and season to taste. If sauce is thinner, return to heat and reduce a little further.

Slice the lamb and spoon a little of the sauce over each serving. Serve the remainder in a sauce boat.

Coat 'n rack of lamb

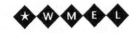

Required number of racks of lamb (rack of 3 per person)
60 g/2 oz ground rice
2 cloves garlic crushed
60 g/2 oz fresh flat-leaf parsley, chopped
60 g/2 oz fresh coriander, chopped
1½ rings canned pineapple, drained and crushed
1–2 tbsp sunflower oil
pinch salt

In a bowl, combine the ground rice, garlic, parsley, coriander, pineapple, oil and seasoning to taste. Mix well.

Wrap a piece of tin foil around the bones of the lamb. Lay the racks of lamb in a non-metallic dish, backs uppermost. Press the mixture firmly on to the backs of the racks.

Cover and refrigerate for several hours.

Transfer the lamb to suitable oven dish, cover and bake for the required time in a moderate oven.

Note: Adding 2–3 tbsp of water in the bottom of the dish will steam in the cooking and keep the lamb moist.

Lamb meatballs with yoghurt dressing

Serves 3–4

450 g/1 lb minced lamb
1 tbsp fresh parsley, chopped
1 egg yolk
¼ tsp cinnamon
¼ tsp cumin
¼ tsp garam masala
pinch paprika
vegetable oil
gram or wheat-free flour

Dressing:
soya yoghurt
1 clove garlic, crushed
½ tsp rice vinegar
2 tsp fresh chopped mint
1 tsp caster sugar (or sweetener)

Put the lamb, parsley, spices and egg yolk in a bowl and combine well. With floured hands, shape spoonfuls of mixture into balls.

Heat a little oil in a pan or wok, add the meatballs and fry, turning regularly, until cooked and evenly browned.

Combine all the dressing ingredients and mix well.

Place a portion of the meatballs on a plate. Place a small dish of yoghurt dressing on the side of plate.

Serve with a rice dish.

Grilled lamb chops with apple and mint butter

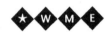

Serves 6–8

6–8 lamb chops
oil for brushing
60 g/2 oz dairy-free margarine
1 tbsp cooked eating apple, well drained of juice
2 tsp mint leaves, chopped
spikes of chives

Cream the margarine until soft and gently mix in the cooked apple and chopped mint.

Place on a piece of baking parchment and chill in the coldest part of the fridge for 30 minutes.

Remove from the fridge, shape into a roll, wrap in the parchment and return to the coldest part of the fridge to chill well.

Brush the chops with the oil, and grill, turning once and brushing again until cooked.

Serve with two slices of the chilled apple mint topping and garnish with chives, accompanied with baked potato and steamed vegetables.

Lancashire hotpot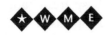
Serves 4

2 large carrots, chopped
1 large leek
2 sticks celery, chopped and equal amount of swede, chopped
170 g/6 oz lentils, soaked and prepared
1 tbsp tomato purée
675 g/1½ lbs lean lamb, cubed
a little wheat- and corn-free flour
salt and pepper
600 ml/1 pint of lamb or vegetable stock (see pages 190–191)
a pinch rosemary
1 large sweet potato, scrubbed and boiled for about 6 minutes

Place all the chopped vegetables in a large casserole. Mix the tomato purée into the stock, season and pour over the vegetables.

Season the flour and coat the lamb well. Place the lamb on top of the vegetables, cover and put into a moderate oven. Cook for 2–2½ hours. Check occasionally to add more stock if necessary.

Remove from the oven. Slice the sweet potato very thinly and layer over the top of the lamb. Lightly brush with oil.

Return to the oven uncovered until the potatoes are cooked and lightly browned on top.

Rissoles
Serves 4

450 g/1 lb minced lamb

170 g/6 oz red lentils, washed, brought to the boil and
   simmered for 20 minutes
170 g/6 oz leeks, finely chopped
85–115 g/3–4 oz suitable bread crumbs, wheat-free
60–85 g/2–3 oz wheat-free porridge flakes, lightly toasted
   and then ground
1 tbsp fresh parsley, chopped
1 tbsp fresh coriander, chopped
1 large egg, lightly beaten
85 g/3 oz tofu
salt and pepper
a little wheat-free flour

Place all the ingredients except the flour into a food processor.
Process gently to mix all the ingredients together.

   Using floured hands, shape spoonfuls of the mixture into
cakes. Well oil a heavy-bottomed frying pan or wok. Add the
rissoles and fry, turning once, until cooked through and golden
brown.

Baked stuffed marrow

Serves 3–4

1 small marrow
170 g/6 oz minced lamb
1–2 tbsp apple purée
85 g/3 oz cooked rice
2 tbsp sunflower oil (preferably 'buttery' variety
salt and pepper
1 tbsp celery, chopped
1–2 tsp rosemary
1 egg lightly beaten
1 tbsp chopped parsley
1 large tomato
a few poppy seeds

Wash and peel the marrow and cut into 5 cm/2 in rings.
Gently scoop out the seeds. Blanch the marrow rings in salted
boiling water for 5 minutes. Remove and drain.

Heat 1 tbsp oil in a pan, add the lamb, seal and cook
through until meat is tender.

Remove from heat. Add the apple purée, rice, celery, rosemary, parsley, egg and seasoning and mix well to bind.

Fill the marrow rings generously, top with slices of tomato
and drizzle over a little oil. Place in a greased baking dish,
cover and bake for 25–30 minutes in a moderate oven. Remove
cover to brush tops with oil, sprinkle with a few poppy seeds
and return to the oven for about 10 minutes to crisp.

Herb marinade for lamb (or pork)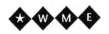

Serves 6

150 ml/¼ pint apple juice
2 tbsp rice wine vinegar
2 tbsp white grape juice
2 tbsp olive oil
2 tbsp fresh parsley, chopped
1 tsp dried mixed herbs
salt and freshly ground black pepper

Mix all the ingredients together in a bowl or screw-topped
jar. When required, pour over the meat, cover and leave for
at least 6 hours, turning the meat occasionally.

Pork

Cheat's chow mein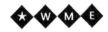

Serves 4

450 g/1 lb pork pieces
170 g/6 oz prawns
4 large chestnut mushrooms, cut into matchsticks
85–115 g/3–4 oz bean sprouts
small green pepper
2 large carrots, cut into batons
salt and black pepper
2 tbsp sunflower oil
300 ml/½ pint chicken stock (see page 190)
1 tsp Mirrin (Japanese sweet rice seasoning) or sweet rice
  vinegar available from good health food shops
8 oz rice noodles

Cook the noodles as directed and keep warm.

Heat the oil in a pan or wok, add the carrots and green pepper and stir fry for 2–3 minutes. Add the pork and mushrooms and stir fry for 6–8 minutes. Add the bean sprouts and salt and pepper to taste and continue to stir fry for 1½–2 minutes.

Add the stock and Mirrin and cook for a further 1½ minutes. Stir in the prawns and leave for 1½ minutes. Refresh noodles with boiling water, pour into a serving dish and spoon the chow mein on top.

Baked gammon pot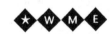

Serves 4–6

1.5 kg/3 lb approx gammon joint
1 stick celery, chopped
1 large carrot, chopped
1 leek, sliced

1 tbsp parsley
1 bay-leaf
2 or 3 whole cloves garlic
1 tsp demerara sugar

Put the gammon in a bowl, cover with cold water and leave to soak for 2–4 hours or overnight. Rinse in fresh cold water, place in a saucepan, cover with cold water and bring to the boil. Allow to boil for 2 minutes, drain, rinse with cold water and put in a casserole.

Add the vegetables, parsley, bay-leaf, garlic and sugar. Cover with water, place in the oven and bake at 160°C/325°F/Gas Mark 3 for 20 minutes per 450 g/lb plus 20 minutes, or until cooked.

Remove from the oven, keep covered and leave to rest in a warm place for 20 minutes. Serve hot or cold.

Somerset pork casserole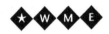

Serves 4

4 pork fillets or 565 g/1¼ lb pork pieces
1 tbsp sunflower oil
1 medium leek, chopped
2 sticks celery, chopped
170 ml/6 fl oz apple juice or white grape juice
2–3 tbsp water
generous pinch dried sage or, preferably, 1 tsp fresh sage, chopped
1 clove garlic, crushed
salt and pepper
30 g/1 oz arrowroot
2 tbsp soya cream

Heat the oil in a pan, add the fillets or pieces of pork and sauté until sealed and beginning to brown. Remove to a casserole. Cook the leek and celery in the pan in the same oil for 4–5 minutes until beginning to soften, but do not allow to brown. Remove and add to the casserole.

Pour the water and apple or grape juice into the pan. Add the sage and garlic, season to taste and bring to the boil. Remove from the heat.

Mix the arrowroot with a little water. Add 2 tbsp of hot stock from the pan and mix well, then pour back into the pan. Return to the heat and simmer for 2 minutes, until the liquid has thickened.

Pour into the casserole and bake at 180°C/350°F/Gas Mark 4 for 40–45 minutes. Remove from the oven, stir in the cream and serve.

Chilli pork ragout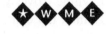

Serves 4

450 g/1 lb pork pieces
2 tbsp sunflower oil
225–280 g/8–10 oz (dry weight) long-grain rice, cooked
140 g/5 oz celery, finely chopped
170 g/6 oz red kidney beans, cooked
1 small green pepper, cut into chunks
1 small red pepper, cut into chunks
3 spikes chives, chopped
½ tsp dried basil
½ tsp ground ginger
½ tsp turmeric
½ tsp chilli powder, or to taste
170 ml/6 fl oz good stock (see page 190)
salt and pepper

In a large pan or wok, heat the oil and sauté the pork pieces until lightly golden and just tender. Remove from the pan and keep warm.

In the same pan, cook the celery, beans, peppers, chives, spices and stock over a gentle heat until the vegetables are just tender. Return the pork to the pan and cook until it is heated through and the moisture is absorbed.

Pour boiling water through the rice to warm and serve with the chilli ragout.

Orchard pork chops

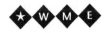

Serves 2

2 pork chops, trimmed and seasoned
½ large cooking apple or 1 medium apple, peeled, cored and chopped
1 pear, peeled, cored and chopped
2 whole cloves garlic
1 small tsp demerara sugar
salt

Line an ovenproof dish with tin foil, leaving enough on the sides to fold over. Lay the chops in the dish.

Put the apple and pear in a saucepan adding the sugar and a little water. Cook over a medium heat until the fruit is pulped. Remove from heat and strain.

Add the juice to the chops, sprinkle with cloves and add a little water and a pinch of salt. Fold the foil over the chops and bake at 180°C/350°F/Gas Mark 4 for 30–40 minutes.

Pork and pineapple grill

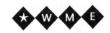

Serves 4

4 lean pork chops
1 tbsp sunflower oil
340 g/12 oz spinach, fresh or frozen
salt and pepper
4 pineapple rings (one small tin)
1 dessertspoon pine nuts, toasted

1 dessertspoon sunflower seeds, toasted
pinch nutmeg

Heat the grill pan, brush both sides of the chops with oil,
season and place under a moderate grill. Grill for 8–10
minutes, depending on the thickness of the meat, brushing
often with oil. Turn the chops and cook for a further 8 minutes.
Remove from the pan and keep warm.

Drain the pineapple, brush with oil and grill both sides
until lightly golden. Put the spinach in a hot pan with 2 tsp
of oil and a pinch of nutmeg. Sweat, stirring continuously,
for 2–3 minutes, until the spinach is wilting,

Remove from the pan and put in the base of warm dish.
Lay the pork chops on top, place a pineapple ring on each
chop and sprinkle toasted nuts and seeds over the whole
dish.

Pan-fried pork with herb sauce

Serves 4

4 lean pork steaks
2 tbsp olive oil
2 cloves garlic, thinly sliced
3 tbsp roughly chopped oregano
small sprig of lemon thyme
115 ml/4 fl oz balsamic vinegar
340 g/12 oz chicken or vegetable stock (see pages 190–191)

Cover the steaks with two sheets of cling film and batter until
1 cm/½ in thick.

Heat the oil in a large frying pan, add the garlic and cook
until it begins to sizzle. Remove and keep warm. Season the
steaks both sides, coat with the herbs and place in the pan.
Cook for approximately 6 minutes, turning once. When
cooked, remove to a plate and keep warm.

Pour the vinegar into the pan and heat until it bubbles.

Scrape up any bits from the pan and continue to bubble until reduced and syrupy.

Pour the sauce over the steaks, scatter with the reserved garlic and serve with crushed potatoes and vegetables.

Pork and cucumber nutty stir fry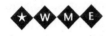

Serves 4

450 g/1 lb lean pork escalopes, cut into strips
1 cucumber, deseeded and cut into thin strips
115 g/4 oz fresh bean sprouts
2 tbsp olive oil or other suitable
1 tsp grated fresh ginger
2 tbsp fresh chives, chopped
1 tbsp sesame seeds, toasted
1–1½ tbsp pine nuts, toasted
2 tsp arrowroot
1 tbsp fresh pineapple juice
150 ml/¼ pint chicken stock (see page 190)

Heat the oil in a large frying pan or wok and fry the pork strips over a high heat for 2–3 minutes until lightly browned. Add the ginger, cucumber and beansprouts, and stir for 2–3 minutes. Add the sesame seeds and pine nuts and toss in the pan for 1 minute.

Mix the arrowroot with pineapple juice. Add the stock to the pan and heat. Gently blend in the arrowroot mixture, bring to the boil, remove from heat and serve with wheat-free pasta or rice.

Pork and sweet potato gratin

Serves 2–3

900 g/2 lb sweet potatoes, peeled and chopped
450g/1 lb cabbage, finely shredded

1 tbsp olive oil
2 tbsp chives, chopped
225 g/8 oz cooked pork, cut into chunks (a good way to use
    up leftovers from joints)
30 g/1 oz pure dairy-free margarine
½ 450 g tub garlic and herb toffutti

Cook the sweet potatoes for 15 minutes, add the shredded
cabbage and cook for a further 4 minutes, then remove from
the heat.

Heat the oil in a frying pan or wok, stir in the pork and
chives until heated through. Keep warm.

Grease a large, shallow ovenproof dish. Drain the vegetables and mash with the margarine, seasoning to taste. Spoon
the vegetables over the base of the dish. Scatter over the pork
and chives. Roughly spread over the toffutti, then place under
a hot grill until the toffutti is starting to bubble.

Pork with pine nuts

Serves 3–4

450 g/1 lb pork fillet
2 tbsp olive oil
30 g/1 oz pine nuts toasted
1 tbsp sweet rice wine vinegar
1 tbsp clear honey
2 tbsp fresh parsley, chopped
a little wheat- and corn-free flour
salt and pepper

Season the flour. Cut the pork into cubes and coat in the
flour. Heat half the olive oil in a pan or wok, add the pork
and cook for 3–4 minutes. Remove to a warm dish.

Add the remaining oil, pine nuts, rice wine vinegar and
honey and mix together, then heat until bubbling, stirring
continuously. Lower the heat to simmer, return the pork to

the pan, fold in the parsley and cook until the pork cubes are tender.

Serve with wheat-free pasta or crushed potatoes and green vegetables.

If desired, 1 tbsp of white pure grape juice can be added to the sauce.

Pork provençal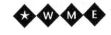

Serves 3–4

450 g/1 lb thick pork escalopes, cut into strips
1 clove garlic, crushed
1 red pepper, or mixture of red, yellow, orange peppers, deseeded and finely chopped
½ small aubergine, salted and rinsed
450 g/1 lb tomatoes
60 g/2 oz dairy-free margarine
1 tbsp olive oil
1 tbsp tomato purée
1 tbsp chopped fresh basil
1 tbsp chopped fresh chives

Melt the margarine in the pan. Add the oil and pork strips and cook for 2 minutes, stirring and turning until lightly golden. Remove from the pan to a warmed dish and keep warm.

Add the garlic and peppers to the pan and cook until beginning to soften. Add the tomatoes, tomato purée, basil and chives and 150 ml /¼ pint water. Bring the contents of pan to the boil, stirring occasionally. Return the pork to the pan and simmer, partially covered, for 15 minutes or until pork is cooked. Serve with wheat-free pasta or rice.

Crispy pork steaks

Serves 4

4 pork steaks
salt and pepper
115 g/4 oz wheat-free dried breadcrumbs or flaked rice,
   toasted and coarsely ground
1–2 tbsp wheat-free flour
1 tsp wheat-free English mustard powder
1 egg, beaten
1 tsp dried parsley
½ tsp dried thyme
¼ tsp dried rosemary or 1 tsp dried oregano
4 tbsp sunflower oil

Cover the steaks with greaseproof paper and flatten to equal thickness.

On a large platter, mix the crumbs or flaked rice with herbs and seasoning. Mix the flour and mustard on another plate. Add 1 tbsp oil to the beaten egg. Coat the steaks well in the flour mix and then in the egg mixture, press into the herbed crumbs until well coated.

Heat the remaining oil in a large pan and fry the steaks for 4–5 minutes each side, or until crisp and golden.

Serve with crushed new potatoes and roasted vegetables.

Apple and mustard pork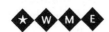

Serves 4

4 lean pork loin steaks
4–6 spikes of chives, according to taste, finely chopped
1 tbsp pure wheat- and corn-free mustard
6 tbsp apple sauce (check ingredients)
300 ml/½ pint vegetable stock (see page 190)
fresh mint to garnish

Season the steaks on both sides with the salt and pepper. Heat 2 tbsp olive oil in a non-stick frying pan, add the steaks and fry for 2 minutes each side or until golden brown. Transfer to a warmed plate.

Add the chives to the pan, stir in the mustard mixed with the apple sauce and stock, and bring to the boil. Reduce to a low simmer and return the steaks to the pan. Continue to simmer gently in the sauce, turning once, until evenly cooked.

Pork steaks with apple and green pepper

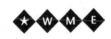

Serves 4

2 tsp sunflower oil
4 lean pork steaks cut about 1 cm/½ in thick
1 clove garlic, peeled and crushed
115 g/4 oz chestnut mushrooms, wiped and sliced
1 small green pepper, de-seeded and chopped
1 red eating apple, cored and sliced
salt and freshly ground black pepper

Heat the oil in a large frying pan and cook the steaks for 15 minutes over a moderate heat, turning once. Remove from pan and keep warm. Add the garlic, mushrooms, apple and pepper to the pan and cook over a medium heat for about 2–3 minutes. Pour apple juice over and boil until reduced and slightly thickened. Season to taste.

Pour over steaks and serve.

Barbecue spare ribs

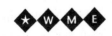

Serves 1–2

900 g/2 lb lean pork spare ribs
2 tbsp fresh chives, chopped
1 clove garlic, peeled and crushed

3 tbsp wheat-free soy sauce
2 tbsp olive oil
3 tbsp apple juice with 2 tsp of sweet rice wine vinegar
3 tbsp tomato purée
1 tbsp soft brown sugar or clear honey
1 tbsp five spice powder
salt and ground black pepper

Put the spare ribs in a shallow dish. Mix the remaining ingredients together in a bowl, until smooth, and pour over the meat. Cover and leave in a cool place turning regularly for 6 hours.

Grill or barbecue over a moderate heat, turning frequently, or bake in the oven at 200°C/400°F/ Gas Mark 6 until juices run clear when meat near bone is tested with a skewer.

Chinese stir fry

Serves 4

1 tbsp oil
405 g/1 lb lean pork, cut into thin strips
2 cloves garlic, crushed
1 tbsp chives, chopped
115 g/4 oz mushrooms, wiped and sliced
1 red pepper, de-seeded and cut into strips
340 g/12 oz pineapple cubes, drained (if canned)
170 g/6 oz water chestnuts, drained and sliced
225–255 g/8–9 oz bean sprouts
salt and black pepper
2 tbsp balsamic vinegar
1 tsp ground cumin

Heat the oil in a wok. Add the pork and garlic and cook over a high heat, stirring continuously, for 5–6 minutes. Add all the remaining ingredients and cook, still stirring, for a further 5 minutes. Serve hot with fried rice.

Stocks, dressings, sauces and chutney

Stock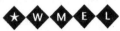

If you make your own stock you can be sure that it is appropriate for your allowed diet. It is also inexpensive, and is to hand whenever you need it.

The basic ingredients for a good stock are:

1 large carrot
1 leek
1 or 2 sticks celery
bouquet garni

To this add fish bones, chicken carcass or beef bones. Cover with water, add salt and pepper and bring to the boil. Skim off any scum that may appear, reduce to the lowest heat and allow the pot to simmer slowly for 2–3 hours. Do not be tempted to stir the contents of the pan – this would give you a cloudy stock.

Turn off the heat, remove the pan from the cooker and leave the stock to rest until just warm. Strain to remove vegetables, bones and bouquet garni. Allow to become cold and skim off any fat that may have settled. Pour into suitable containers and freeze.

Vegetable stock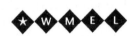

The most economical way of making vegetable stock is to save usable vegetable trimmings when preparing vegetables for meals. Put them into a covered tub in the refrigerator. They will keep for a couple of days.

Rinse the vegetables/trimmings, put them in a pan with a handful of fresh mixed herbs and cover with salted water. Bring to the boil and simmer for 1–1½ hours. Strain the liquid from the vegetables and leave to cool. Spoon into suitable containers and freeze.

For convenience, you can use some of the commercial alternatives that are available. Supermarkets produce their own fresh stocks, although chicken stock tends to be the only one suitable for the exclusion diet (check ingredients carefully). Some stock cubes and powders are available from health-food shops that are wheat-, dairy- and yeast-free.

Curry salad dressing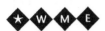

225 ml/8 fl oz soya yoghurt
2 tsp korma curry powder (check ingredients carefully)
2 level tsp tomato purée
60 ml/2 fl oz pineapple juice
Mix all the ingredients together thoroughly until blended. Keep refrigerated.

Mushroom sauce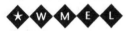

225 g/8 oz mushrooms, wiped and chopped
30 g/1 oz sunflower oil or dairy-free margarine
280–340 g/10–12 oz beef or chicken stock (see page 190)
1 heaped tsp fresh mixed herbs, finely chopped
little arrowroot if necessary
salt and pepper

Heat the oil in a pan or wok, add the mushrooms and cook for 2–3 minutes. Add the stock and herbs, bring to the boil and lower the heat to a simmer for 5–6 minutes.

Set aside 1 tsp of chopped mushrooms, transfer remaining contents to liquidizer and blend.

Return to the pan and add the reserved mushrooms. Reheat, thickening with a little arrowroot if necessary.

Savoury white sauce

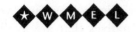

300 ml/½ pint soya milk
15 g/½ oz dairy-free margarine
salt
4–6 black peppercorns
2 tsp wheat-free Dijon mustard (or 2 tbsp fresh chives or
    parsley, chopped)
little arrowroot to thicken
small bay-leaf

Put the milk, margarine, salt to taste, black peppercorns, and
bay-leaf in a saucepan. Heat over a very low heat until hot,
but not boiling.

Remove from the heat and leave to infuse for 30 minutes.
Remove the bay-leaf and peppercorns and stir in the Dijon
mustard or herbs. Mix the arrowroot with a little cold soya
milk, add 2 tbsp warm soya milk and return to the saucepan.

Mix well and return to the heat. Bring to the boil, stirring, then simmer for 2 minutes.

Herb dressing

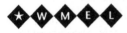

170–280 ml/6–10 fl oz light olive oil, depending on amount
    you wish to make
2–3 tbsp apple juice or white grape juice
2 tbsp fresh chives, chopped
2 tbsp fresh parsley, chopped
1 tbsp fresh dill, chopped
salt to taste

Add the herbs to the juice and whisk well together. Gradually
add the oil, drop by drop, whisking continuously. Transfer
to a screw-top container and refrigerate until required.

Mint and cucumber yogurt sauce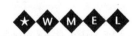

300 ml/½ pint soya yoghurt
2 tsp fresh chives, finely chopped
1 tbsp fresh mint leaves, chopped
1 heaped tbsp cucumber, chopped
salt to taste

Whisk all the ingredients together in a bowl and refrigerate until needed.
     This sauce is ideal for curries.

Hasty tomato and mushroom sauce

1 stick celery, chopped
1–2 tbsp olive oil
115 g/4 oz mushrooms, sliced
400 g/14 oz jar of sieved or tinned tomatoes, drained
2 tbsp tomato purée
2 tsp chives, chopped
pinch each oregano, thyme and basil
1 small bay-leaf
salt and pepper

Cook the celery in the oil for 2–3 minutes, then add the mushrooms, tomatoes, purée, herbs and seasoning. Simmer on a very low heat for 10 minutes. Remove the bay-leaf, and serve as required.

Lentil apple sauce

115 g/4 oz lentils, washed, soaked and ready to cook
850 ml/1½ pints vegetable stock (see page 190)
garni of chives, thyme and a small bay-leaf
1–2 tbsp sunflower oil
2 large carrots, chopped
1 large stick celery, finely sliced

1 large Cox's apple (a Bramley can be used), peeled, cored
   and chopped
salt and pepper

Cook the lentils in the stock for 30–40 minutes with the herb
garni. Heat the oil in a frying pan, add the carrots and celery
and cook for about 5 minutes over a low heat. Then add the
apple.

   Continue cooking until the carrots and celery are cooked.
Transfer to a blender, add the lentils and blend well. Season
to taste with salt and pepper.

   Alternatively, run the sauce through a sieve until smooth.

Mayonnaise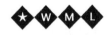

2 large egg yolks
a pinch salt
½ tsp wheat-free Dijon mustard
2 tbsp creamed coconut
150 ml/¼ pint light olive oil

Whisk the egg yolks with the salt, Dijon mustard and creamed
coconut. When smooth, add the olive oil just 2–3 drops at a
time. Chill until required.

Hollandaise sauce

4 egg yolks
115 ml/4 fl oz sunflower oil (preferably 'buttery' variety)
1 tbsp white grape juice
salt and pepper
1 tbsp soya cream
Put the egg yolks, grape juice and seasoning into a blender,
turn on. Warm the buttery oil and, when hot but not coloured,
pour into the blender in a thin stream. The mixture should

thicken. Process until smooth. Add the cream very slowly down blender tunnel, still processing.

You should have a thick golden sauce. Keep warm over a pan of hot water until ready to serve. A damp greaseproof paper lid over the top will prevent it drying out.

Basil tomato sauce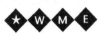

450 g/1 lb tomatoes, skinned, seeded and chopped
2 level tbsp tomato purée
6 tbsp chicken stock (see page 190)
salt and pepper to taste
1 tbsp fresh parsley, finely chopped
few drops of pure basil oil

Put all the ingredients in a saucepan and cook through over a medium heat until well blended and thickened slightly. Remove from heat and add parsley and basil oil. (Fresh basil leaves, torn, can be used instead of oil.)

This sauce can be used for grilled or baked fish and also in chicken and turkey dishes.

Mustard sauce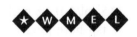

30 g/1 oz dairy-free margarine or sunflower oil (preferably 'buttery' variety)
2 heaped tsp wheat- and corn-free Dijon mustard
1 tsp wheat- and corn-free Worcester sauce
170 g/6 oz soya cream
salt and pepper

Heat the margarine or oil, add the mustard, Worcester sauce and soya cream, and season to taste.

Heat gently until the sauce just reaches boiling point, stirring continuously.

Sweet and sour sauce

1 can vegetable juice
2 tsp tomato purée
5 tbsp apple or pineapple juice
1 tbsp rice vinegar
salt and pepper
1 tbsp demerara sugar
a little arrowroot to thicken

Put all the ingredients except the arrowroot into a small heavy-based pan. Heat gently, stirring until the sugar has dissolved and the liquid is smooth.

Thicken with a little arrowroot, bring to the boil and then simmer for 2 minutes.

Mango chutney

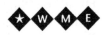

1½ kg/3 ½ lb ripe mango, peeled and chopped
½ tsp salt
115 g/4 oz raisins, chopped
500 ml/18 fl oz sweet rice wine vinegar
115 ml/4 fl oz molasses or equal amount of apricot jam
½ tsp pure ginger

Mix the chopped mangoes and salt in a bowl, add the chopped raisins, vinegar, molasses (or jam) and ginger.

Simmer over a gentle heat until thick and creamy. While still hot, pour into clean sterile jars with airtight lids and seal immediately.

Small amounts of this chutney can be made as required and stored in the fridge when cold.

Desserts

Gingered pears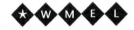

Serves 6

6 firm pears
225 ml/8 fl oz white grape juice
25 mm/1 in piece of fresh ginger, peeled and cut into three
   pieces
little soya cream
chopped stem ginger to garnish

Peel the pears, leaving the stems on, and slice across the
bottoms so that the pears stand up.

Place the pears in a saucepan, pour over the grape juice
and add the ginger. Cover and cook over a low heat until the
pears are just tender. Remove from the heat and leave to cool.

To serve, remove the ginger and place the pears in individual dishes, spooning a little juice over them. Pour a little
soya cream around the base of each pear and sprinkle a little
chopped stem ginger into the cream.

Apple and sultana brûlée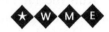

Serves 2

3 medium apples, peeled, cored and chopped
85 g/3 oz sultanas
brown sugar to taste
2 tbsp water
2 x 120 g/4 oz cartons soya yoghurt
brown sugar

Put the apples, sugar and water in a pan and poach until the
apples are tender. Stir in the sultanas and poach for a further
5 minutes, until the liquid has reduced.

Divide the fruit between two individual dishes and empty a carton of yoghurt into each dish. Sprinkle a layer of brown sugar over the top and place under a hot grill until the sugar caramelizes.

The brûlée can be served on its own or with a piece of shortbread (see page 218).

Pear and raspberry crumble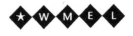

Serves 4

2 medium pears, peeled, cored and sliced
115 g/4 oz raspberries, washed
little sugar if necessary

Crumble topping:
115 g/4 oz high-fibre flour mix (see page 213)
60 g/2 oz dairy-free margarine
40 g/1½ oz caster sugar
1 tsp cinnamon

Poach the fruit until it begins to soften, adding sugar if required, then place in a basin or ovenproof dish.

Rub the fat into the flour to a breadcrumb consistency. Stir in the sugar and cinnamon until evenly mixed and spoon over the fruit.

Bake for 20–25 minutes, or until golden brown, at 180°C/ 350°F/Gas Mark 4.

Banana and sultana pudding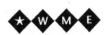

Serves 2

600 ml/1 pint soya milk
60 g/2 oz caster sugar
60 g/2 oz flaked rice
60 g/2 oz sultanas

pinch cinnamon
2 bananas
2 heaped tbsp demerara sugar

Put the milk, sugar, rice, sultanas and cinnamon in a saucepan. Bring slowly to the boil, stirring frequently. Lower the heat and simmer for 12–15 minutes, until thick.

Pour into a suitable heat-proof dish. Slice the bananas thinly and lay over the top. Cover with a thick layer of sugar. Brown under the grill.

Serve hot or cold with a little soya cream if wished.

Moreish pear and apricot quickie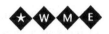

Serves 4

280 g/10 oz pears, peeled, cored and sliced
225 g/8 oz dried, ready-to-eat apricots, halved
225 ml/8 fl oz water
1 large tbsp honey
pinch cinnamon
pinch ground cloves (optional)
1½ heaped tbsp brown sugar
1 tbsp pine nuts

Put the pears, apricots, water, honey and spices in a saucepan over a gentle heat and poach until the fruit is tender.

Remove the fruit to a suitable ovenproof dish, increase the heat and boil the poaching liquid until thick and syrupy. Pour over the fruit, spoon the sugar over the top and sprinkle with pine nuts. Place under a hot grill until the sugar has caramelized and the pine nuts are toasted.

Pear condé

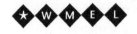

Serves 4

600 ml/1 pint soya milk
30 g/1 oz caster sugar
85 g/3 oz pudding rice, washed
few drops vanilla essence
8 pear halves, poached until tender, or canned in natural
    juices
4 tbsp apricot jam
120 g/4 oz carton soya yoghurt

Put the milk, sugar, rice and vanilla essence in an ovenproof dish
and bake in a slow oven for 1½–2 hours, stirring occasionally.

When the rice is cooked and most of the milk has been
absorbed, remove, leave until cool, then chill in the refrigerator.

Divide the rice pudding between four bowls and lay the
pear halves on top, cut side down. Warm the apricot jam and
use it to brush the pears and rice well.

Spoon over a thickish topping of soya yoghurt, make a
swirl in the yoghurt with a fork and serve.

Simply super sweet

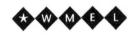

Serves 1

mixture of fresh mango, pineapple and papaya sliced (to individual taste)
sunflower oil (preferably 'buttery' variety)
ground ginger to taste
few drops vanilla essence

Heat the grill to medium-high, line the grill pan with tin foil
and lay the fruit in layers on the foil.

Pour a little sunflower oil into a small bowl. Add 2–3 drops
of vanilla essence. Brush well over fruit and sprinkle with
ground ginger.

Place under the grill until bubbling and lightly golden. Then turn the fruit over and repeat on the other side.

Serve with soya yoghurt or, for a special treat, liquidize a slice of ripe melon and add 1 tsp medium-sweet white wine to serve with it as a sauce.

Taste of Jamaica

Serves 4

wheat-free pastry using 225 g/8 oz flour mix (see page 212)
2 bananas, sliced
½ large mango, chopped
115 g/4 oz golden syrup
60 g/2 oz wheat-free breadcrumbs or wheat-free sponge cake crumbs (see pages 214, 228)
½ tsp ground ginger

Line a greased 18–20 cm/7–8 inch pie plate with the pastry, reserving enough to make a top. Cover the base with a mixture of mango and banana.

Stir the crumbs and ground ginger into the golden syrup and spoon over the fruit. Roll out the remaining pastry and cover the pie.

Bake at 180°C/350°F/Gas Mark 4 for 25–30 minutes, or until the pastry is cooked and the top is golden brown. This dessert may take a little effort, but it is certainly worth it!

Pancake mixture

Serves 4

115 g/4 oz flour mix (see page 212)
pinch salt
1 egg
85 ml/3 fl oz soya milk plus 85 ml/3 fl oz water
1 tbsp sunflower oil

Sift the flour and salt together in a bowl. Make a well in the centre, put in the egg and a little of the milk and beat really well until smoothly blended. Gradually add the remaining liquid until you have a smooth batter of a creamy consistency. Leave in a cool place for 20 minutes. Add 1 tbsp oil and beat for 2 minutes, then leave to rest for 10 minutes.

Heat the remaining oil in a frying pan. When very hot, whisk the batter and pour in the required amount. Cook over a fairly high heat. When the edges are curling and golden, turn the pancake and cook the remaining batter in the same way.

The pancakes can be used for either sweet or savoury fillings.

Summer pudding

Serves 6

sponge mixture made with 170 g/6 oz flour mix and wheat-free baking powder (see pages 212, 214)
1 large cooking apple, peeled, cored and chopped
450 g/1 lb red fruit, e.g. plums, berries
sugar to taste
115 ml/4 fl oz water

Grease and line a swiss-roll tin, pour in the sponge mixture and bake. Remove from the oven and cool.

Meanwhile, put the apple in a saucepan with some sugar and the water and cook for 15–20 minutes. Add the other fruit and continue cooking until all the fruit is soft. Remove from the heat and set aside to cool.

Cut two-thirds of the sponge into wedges and line a glass or ceramic basin. Pour in the fruit mixture and cut the remainder of the sponge to fit the top as a lid. Place a saucer or plate on top and weigh it down. Leave in the refrigerator overnight.

Serve with soya cream or soya yoghurt.

Bread pudding

Serves 6

wheat-free bread loaf using 450 g/1 lb flour mix (see page
    212)
300 ml/½ pint soya milk
1 large egg, beaten
115 g/4 oz sugar, preferably moist brown sugar
225 g/8 oz dried fruit, mixed
1 tsp mixed spice
¼ tsp cinnamon

Cut the bread into cubes and soak in the milk until the liquid
has been absorbed. Stir to make sure there are no lumps.

Add all the remaining ingredients, mixing well to combine.
The mixture should not be too wet.

Spoon into a greased and lined 5 cm/2 in deep rectangular
cake tin (18–20 cm/7–8 inch square). Sprinkle a mixture of
brown sugar and cinnamon over the top and bake at
180°C/350°F/Gas Mark 4 for 1–1¼ hours, or until cooked
and firm to the touch.

Baked banana sponge

Serves 4

115 g/4 oz high-fibre flour mix plus 1 tsp wheat-free baking
    powder sifted together (see pages 213, 214)
85 g/3 oz dairy-free margarine
60 g/2 oz caster sugar
vanilla essence
2 small eggs, beaten
2 small bananas, sliced

Cream the margarine and sugar until pale and fluffy. Add a
few drops of vanilla essence to the beaten eggs and stir a little
into the creamed mixture along with 1 tbsp of the flour mix.

Gradually add the remaining egg, sliced bananas and 1 tbsp of flour mix to combine. Fold in the remaining flour mix.

Transfer to greased and lined 450 g/1 lb loaf tin and bake for 20 minutes at 180°C/350°F/Gas Mark 4. Reduce the oven temperature to 160°C/325°F/Gas Mark 3 and bake for a further 20 minutes, or until the sponge is cooked.

Serve with soya custard or soya yoghurt.

Apple cake pudding

Serves 6

225 g/8 oz flour mix plus 2 tsp wheat-free baking powder, sifted together (see pages 212, 214)
115 g/4 oz dairy-free margarine
115 g/4 oz caster sugar
1 egg, beaten
1 medium-large apple, peeled, cored and grated
½ tsp vanilla essence
soya milk
little demerara sugar

Beat the margarine and sugar together until pale and fluffy. Add the beaten egg, vanilla essence and a little flour. Gradually beat in the rest of the flour and add the grated apple. Add sufficient milk to reach a dropping consistency.

Bake at 180°C/350°F/Gas Mark 4 for about 1 hour, or until cooked. This makes an excellent pudding served with soya custard.

Pineapple upside-down pudding

Serves 6

340 g/12 oz pineapple rings, drained
6 glacé cherries

170 g/6 oz flour mix and 1½ tsp wheat-free baking powder
sifted together (see pages 212, 214)
115 g/4 oz dairy-free margarine
60 g/2 oz caster sugar
2 large eggs, beaten
1 tbsp soya milk

Wash the cherries free of their sugar coating, dry and cut into
halves. Dry the pineapple rings using kitchen paper.

Lightly grease and line an 18 cm/7 in cake tin. Put a
pineapple ring in the centre of the tin and arrange the
remaining rings around it. Place a cherry in the centre of each
pineapple ring.

Cream the margarine and sugar until pale and fluffy. Add
the egg a little at a time, adding a spoonful of flour with the
first quantity of egg. Fold in the remaining flour/baking
powder mix. Add the milk to give a dropping consistency.

Spoon the mixture over the pineapple rings, covering them
completely. Bake for 40–45 minutes at 180°C/350°F/Gas Mark
4. Remove from the oven and leave to stand for a few minutes
before turning out onto a dish. Serve hot or cold.

Blackcurrant and tofu whip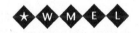

Serves 4–6

450 g/1 lb ripe blackcurrants
sugar to taste
280 g/10 oz tofu

Put the blackcurrants in a pan with a little water and sugar
to taste. Bring to the boil and stew until the blackcurrants
are tender. Leave to cool. Place in a blender with the tofu
and liquidize until smooth. Chill well before serving.

Note: Other fruits such as blackberries or gooseberries can
be substituted for the blackcurrants in this recipe.

Carob ice-cream

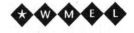

Serves 4–6

60 g/2 oz runny honey
500 ml/18 fl oz soya milk
4 tbsp sunflower oil
¼ tsp salt
60 g/2 oz carob powder

Put all the ingredients in a blender and liquidize until smooth. Pour into a suitable container and freeze for approximately 3 hours, until the mixture begins to set. Beat with a fork, then return to the freezer to firm up for at least 1 hour.

Transfer to the refrigerator 30 minutes before serving, to allow the ice-cream to soften.

Note: This ice-cream can be made with other flavourings besides carob powder, such as puréed fruit.

Apricot mould

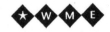

Serves 4

130 g/4½ oz dried apricots
2 tbsp granulated sugar
1 sachet powdered gelatine (about 15 g/½ oz)

Pour boiling water over 100 g/3½ oz of the apricots and leave to soak for several hours. Drain and wash. Stew for 10 minutes, until soft, in 60 ml/2 fl oz water. Sieve to make a purée, then stir in the sugar.

Dissolve the gelatine in 90 ml/3 fl oz very hot water, stirring briskly. Make up to 300 ml/½ pint with cold water, then stir into the apricot mixture.

Arrange the remaining dried apricots on the base of a wetted mould, then carefully pour in the mixture. Allow to set in a refrigerator for 3 hours.

Steamed sponge pudding

Serves 1–2

85 g/3 oz wheat-free flour mix (see page 212)
1 tsp wheat-free baking powder (see page 214)
60 g/2 oz dairy-free margarine
1 egg
1 tbsp jam (flavour of your own choice)

Put the margarine, egg and jam (or sugar) in a bowl and whisk until combined and creamy. Fold in the flour mix with baking powder. Put into a greased suitable dish with lid, or cover with pleated foil, and steam for about 1 hour.

Pear and sultana crunch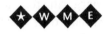

Serves 4

4 pears, peeled, cored and thinly sliced
85 g/3 oz sultanas
115 g/4 oz soft brown sugar
1 tsp cinnamon
¼ tsp ground ginger (optional)
60 ml/2 fl oz white grape juice
140 g/5 oz wheat-, corn- and dairy-free breadcrumbs
85 g/3 oz dairy-free margarine, melted

Mix together the pears and sultanas. In a separate bowl, mix the sugar and spices, remove 4 tbsp and set aside. Stir the remainder into the fruit. Stir in the grape juice.

Mix the breadcrumbs with reserved sugar mixture then stir in the melted margarine.

Lightly press about half the crumb mixture into a greased baking dish, cover with the fruit, sprinkle over remaining crumbs and press down very lightly.

Bake at 180°C/350°F/Gas Mark 4 for 35–40 minutes or until browned and the fruit is soft.

Coconut crumble

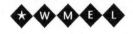

Serves 2–3

60 g/2 oz wheat- and corn-free flour mix (see page 212)
60 g/2 oz toasted rice flakes (or suitable breadcrumbs)
60 g/2 oz desiccated coconut
60 g/2 oz dairy-free margarine
225–280 g/8–10 oz of choice of fruit jam (flavour to comple-
    ment fruit)

Place the fruit in the base of an ovenproof dish. Heat the
jam, adding a little water to thin the consistency slightly. Pour
the jam over the fruit.

Put the flour and rice flakes into a bowl, rub in the
margarine to coarse breadcrumbs and then stir in the coconut.
Spread over the fruit and bake until the top is golden.

The jam makes the fruit sweet and the coconut will lightly
sweeten the topping. Together this should be sweet enough
but additional sugar can be added to the topping, if required.

Mango and apricot delight

Serves 2–3

1 large mango, peeled and flesh cut off the stone
½ 450 g tub of plain toffutti
apricot jam
equal quantity of soya bio yoghurt as to pulped mango

Put the mango and toffutti in a food processor and blend
until smooth.

Put the soya yoghurt in a clean bowl, and mix in spoonfuls of apricot jam to taste.

In a heavy glass tumbler, layer the two mixtures, finishing
with a mango layer.

If allowed, some wheat-free biscuit crumbs sprinkled on
the top makes a crunchy topping

Sweet and spicy crumble

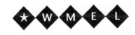

Serves 4

450 g/1 lb ripe pears, peeled, cored and thinly sliced
1 tbsp muscovado sugar or 1 tbsp rice syrup
flesh from 2 mangoes, chopped
1 piece of stem ginger

170 g/6 oz wheat- and corn-free flour
85 g/3 oz dairy-free margarine
85 g/3 oz muscovado sugar or 3 tbsp apricot jam
a few toasted pine nuts

Put the pears into a pan with the sugar (or syrup) and 4 tbsp of water. Simmer gently until the pears are just tender. Remove from the heat and stir in the mangoes and ginger. Transfer to a suitable ovenproof dish and leave to cool.

Put first three ingredients in food processor and pulse until moist crumbs form. Spread over the fruit and bake in oven at 170°C/325°F/Gas Mark 3 for 30–40 minutes until golden brown and crisp on top. Remove from the over, sprinkle the pine nuts over and return to the oven for 5 minutes.

Red fruit condé

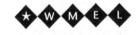

Serves 2

a portion of steamed rice per person
1–2 tbsp red grape juice per portion
1 tbsp mixed red fruit per portion
1 tsp raspberry jam
a little extra red grape juice

Place a portion of rice in a dish and stir in enough red grape juice to sweeten and moisten.

In a non-stick pan, put the fruit, jam and enough juice to cook the fruit and prevent it sticking. Simmer over a gentle heat, stirring continually until the fruit reaches a compôte consistency. If necessary, add a little more jam for sweetness or a little more juice so it is just moist and holding together. Spoon over the top of the rice and serve hot or cold.

Pear and raisin vanilla rice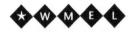

Serves 2

2 oz steamed rice
1–1½ ripe pears per portion, peeled and cored
2–3 drops pure vanilla
a few raisins

Place the rice portions in individual dishes. Put the pears into a blender and liquidize, adding drops of vanilla essence to taste.
    Fold the pear mixture into the rice until well combined. Fold in the raisins and chill.

Strawberry brûlées

Serves 4–6

115 g/4 oz ripe strawberries per person
60 g/2 oz plain toffutti per person
soya bio yoghurt
115 g/4 oz caster sugar
2 tbsp cold water

Crush the strawberries well and mix into a smooth mixture with the toffutti. Spoon into individual ramekins and smooth the top. Add a layer of yoghurt. Chill.
    Put the sugar and water into a small pan, heat slowly to dissolve the sugar stirring constantly. When dissolved, allow to come to the boil, and wait for it to turn a light caramel colour. Remove from the heat and immediately place the base

of the pan into ice-cold water. When the bubbles have subsided, gently pour a little over each dessert. Chill for 1 hour before serving.

Carrot pudding

Serves 4–6

170 g/6 oz dairy-free margarine
115 g/4 oz brown sugar
2 eggs and 1 egg yolk, lightly beaten
2 pinches of cinnamon, nutmeg and allspice
255 g/9 oz grated carrot
255 g/9 oz wheat-free breadcrumbs (see page 214)
1 tbsp wheat-free flour mix (see page 212)

Cream the margarine and sugar, gradually add the eggs and stir in. Add the spices, then fold in the grated carrot and breadcrumbs. Finally fold in the flour.

Bake at 180°C/350°F/Gas Mark 4 for about 30 minutes or until slightly risen and browned in the centre.

As this pudding is spicy, serve with a ripe melon, liquidized, as a sauce.

Baking

Please note, people's ovens vary. It is necessary to know your oven more with baking bread than other dishes. Times and temperatures can vary.

Flour mixes

The gluten-free flour mixes you can buy are usually unsuitable for exclusion diets because they contain wheat starch, corn (or maize) flour, potato flour or a combination of these. They also tend to be expensive as they are prescribable only for those with confirmed Coeliac disease.

Substituting a single alternative flour, e.g. rice flour, for normal wheat flour gives disappointing results when baking because gluten is essential for the light, doughy consistency we associate with bread. However, this characteristic can be mimicked using a combination of flours and a binding agent such as guar gum, xanthan gum or pectin. These flours and binders should all be available from a good health-food shop.

The following mixes are all suitable for wheat-, milk- and egg-free diets. The recipes containing amaranth flour are also suitable for exclusion and LOFFLEX diets. Amaranth flour gives particularly good results. It has a nutty flavour and when mixed with a high-starch grain flour gives a good texture and retains moisture. Unfortunately, it is not as readily available as other flours.

For bread, lighter cakes, pastry and scones choose from recipes A to D. A high-fibre flour mix can be made by adding rice bran to these (recipe E). Recipe F is more suitable for heavier cakes such as fruit cakes and some savoury dishes.

A   225 g/8 oz amaranth flour   ★ W M E L
          450 g/1 lb rice flour
          30 g/1 oz binder (guar gum, xanthan gum or pectin)

B 675 g/1½ lb amaranth flour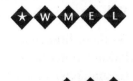
   225 g/8 oz tapioca flour
   30 g/1 oz binder (as above)

C 85 g/3 oz tapioca flour
   60 g/2 oz soya flour
   60 g/2 oz rice flour
   30 g/1 oz cornflour
   15 g/½ oz binder (as above)

D 85 g/3 oz rice flour
   85 g/3 oz tapioca flour
   60 g/2 oz farina (potato starch)
   15 g/½ oz binder (as above)

E For high-fibre flour, add 1 tbsp finely ground rice bran
   to any of the above mixes.

A to E: suitable for bread, lighter cakes, pastry, scones, etc.
Blend all the ingredients together well. Store in an airtight
plastic container.

F 510 g/1 lb 2 oz fine ground
      rice flour   (★ and ⬤ depending on choice
   85 g/4 oz soya flour   of flour mix)
   60 g/2 oz gram flour
   225 g/8 oz polenta or desiccated coconut (this must
      be very finely ground in processor) or 225 g/8 oz
      ground almonds
   30 g/1 oz binder (guar gum, xanthan gum or pectin)

Suitable for heavier cakes such as fruit cakes and some savoury
dishes. Blend all the ingredients together well. Store in an
airtight plastic container. Makes approximately 900 g/2 lb.

Wheat-free baking powder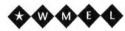

As these flour mixes are very light compared to wheat flour, baking powder works better as a raising agent than yeast. Commercial wheat-free brands are available from health-food shops and some supermarkets, but a cheaper version can be home-made.

170 g/6 oz tapioca or rice flour
200 g/7 oz bicarbonate of soda or potassium bicarbonate
85 g/4 oz cream of tartar
60 g/2 oz tartaric acid

Sieve all the ingredients together and store in an airtight container. Sieve the required amount again just before use.

Soda bread

450 g/16 oz high-fibre flour mix (see page 213)
260 ml/½ pint soya milk
2 egg whites, beaten
¼ tsp salt
1 heaped tsp bicarbonate of soda or potassium bicarbonate
1 heaped tsp cream of tartar
30 g/1 oz sesame seeds

Place the flour, salt, bicarbonate of soda and cream of tartar in a bowl. Add the liquid ingredients, stirring well, until a smooth, thick batter is achieved.

Place the batter in a well-greased 900 g/2 lb loaf tin. Brush the top with oil and sprinkle the sesame seeds on top.

Bake at 180°C/350°F/Gas Mark 4 for 40–45 minutes or until well risen and firm to the touch.

Tomato and basil soda bread

450 g/1 lb high-fibre flour mix (see page 213)
260 ml/½ pint water
2 egg whites, beaten
¼ tsp salt
1 heaped tsp bicarbonate of soda or potassium bicarbonate
1 heaped tsp cream of tartar
60 g/2 oz dried tomatoes
3–4 drops pure basil oil
2 level tbsp fresh basil leaves, torn into pieces
poppy seeds to sprinkle

Soak the dried tomatoes in boiling water for 20 minutes. Drain and dry well and cut into small strips.

Place the flour, salt, bicarbonate of soda and cream of tartar in a bowl. Add the tomato slices and torn basil leaves and stir. Stir the basil oil into the egg and add with water to the dry ingredients. Beat to a smooth but thick batter.

Place the batter in a greased 20 cm/8 in sandwich tin lined with baking paper. Mark a cross in the batter. Brush with oil and sprinkle with poppy seeds.

Bake at 180°C/350°F/Gas Mark 4 for 40–45 minutes or until well risen and firm to the touch.

Chapattis

Makes 10 approx   (★ and L depending on choice of
                                              flour mix)

200 g/7 oz flour mix (see page 212)
30 g/1 oz rice bran
¼ tsp salt
30 g/1 oz dairy-free margarine
150 ml/¼ pint water
sunflower oil for frying

Mix the flour, bran and salt in a bowl. Add the margarine and rub into a breadcrumb consistency. Add water to mix to a stiff dough.

Knead well on a floured board for 5 minutes. Leave to rest for 20 minutes. Divide the dough into ten pieces and roll out each piece into a circle.

Heat the oil in a frying pan and fry each chapatti for 3 minutes, turning frequently. Serve warm.

Sweet potato bread

Makes 16 pieces   (★ and Ⓛ depending on choice of flour mix)

225 g/8 oz sweet potato, scrubbed but not peeled
170 g/6 oz flour mix (see page 212)
pinch salt
pinch nutmeg
pinch cumin
sunflower oil for frying

Cook the potatoes in boiling water for 8–10 minutes. Drain and rinse them in cold water, then remove peel and grate into a bowl.

Add the flour, salt and spices to the potato and mix to a soft dough. Add a little cold water if necessary. Divide the dough into 16 pieces and dust with flour. Roll each piece on a floured board.

Heat the oil in heavy frying pan and shallow fry the bread pieces, a few at a time, for 2–3 minutes. Drain on kitchen paper.

Baker's scones

Makes 6–8 scones (★ and L depending on choice of flour mix)

115 g/4 oz high-fibre flour mix (see page 213)
115 g/4 oz flour mix (see page 212)
or
200 g/7 oz flour mix and
30 g/1 oz pure rice bran

2 tsp wheat-free baking powder (see page 214)
30 g/1 oz caster sugar
60 g/2 oz dairy-free margarine
140 g/5 oz soya milk
½ tsp vanilla essence
pinch salt

Place the flour in a clean bowl, add the salt and baking powder and mix well. Add the margarine and rub in until it resembles fine breadcrumbs. Stir in the sugar.

Add the vanilla essence to the milk and stir. Add to the dry ingredients and mix to a soft but not sticky consistency. Add a little more milk if necessary, but avoid making the mixture too wet.

Flour a board and gently roll the mixture to a good 25 mm/1 in thickness. Cut out the scones and place on a greased baking sheet. Brush the tops with egg or milk if desired.

Bake in the oven for about 10 minutes at 220°C/425°F/Gas Mark 7 or until lightly golden. Leave them to cool, then place them on a wire rack until cold.

Derby scones

Makes 6–8 scones (★ and L depending on choice of flour mix)

225 g/8 oz flour mix (see page 212)
½ tsp salt
2 tsp wheat-free baking powder (see page 214)

30 g/1 oz dairy-free margarine
30 g/1 oz caster sugar
60 g/2 oz sultanas
soya milk to mix, approx 5 tbsp
½ tsp vanilla essence

Sift the flour into a bowl and add the salt and baking powder. Add the margarine and rub into a breadcrumb consistency. Stir in the sugar and sultanas. Stir the vanilla essence into the milk. Add the milk to mix into a soft but not sticky dough.

Roll out on a floured board and cut into 4 cm/1½ in rounds, brush the tops with milk and bake in the oven for 10–12 minutes at 200°C/400°F/Gas Mark 6.

Shortbread

Makes 15–20 pieces   (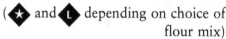 and depending on choice of flour mix)

225 g/8 oz flour mix (see page 212)
115 g/4 oz ground rice
115 g/4 oz caster sugar
225 g/8 oz dairy-free margarine
few drops pure almond essence (optional)

Mix together the flour, rice and sugar. Melt the fat in a saucepan and add the almond essence if using. Add to the dry ingredients and mix together well.

Roll out to 1 cm/½ in thickness, cut into shapes and pinch the edges.

Place on a baking sheet and bake at 180°C/350°F/Gas Mark 4 for about 30 minutes or until lightly golden. Leave to cool on a tray.

Honeyed ginger flapjacks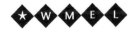

Makes 8–10 fingers

225 g/8 oz millet flakes or rice flakes
140 g/5 oz sunflower oil (preferably 'buttery' variety)
85 g/3 oz light soft brown sugar
2 tbsp clear Mexican honey
⅓–½ tsp ground ginger (to taste)

Preheat the oven to 180°C/350°F/Gas Mark 4.

Pour the oil into a saucepan over a low heat and stir in the sugar, honey, flakes and ginger. Mix very thoroughly. Grease an 18 cm/7 in square shallow baking tin and press in the mixture.

Bake for 20–25 minutes until golden and lightly firm.

Mark into fingers while still hot. Leave in the tin until cold.

Granny's gingerbreads

Makes 8 approx   (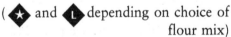 and depending on choice of flour mix)

115 g/4 oz dairy-free margarine
115 g/4 oz caster sugar
115 g/4 oz flour mix (see page 212)
1 tsp wheat-free baking powder (see page 214)
2 tsp ground ginger

Cream the margarine and sugar together until pale. Mix together the flour, baking powder and ginger. Add 1 tbsp of flour mix at a time to the cream mixture to form a stiff dough.

Roll into balls the size of a very small egg and place on a baking sheet, well apart.

Bake on the bottom shelf for 15 minutes at 180°C/350°F/Gas Mark 4. Then leave to cool on a wire tray.

Shortcrust pastry

To cover 20 cm/8 inch pie dish

170 g/6 oz flour mix (see page 212)
¼ tsp salt
60 g/2 oz dairy-free margarine
30 g/1 oz white hard vegetable oil
1 egg, beaten, plus 1 tbsp water

Sift the flour into a bowl and add the salt. Add the fats and rub into a breadcrumb consistency. Add sufficient egg mixture to give a soft, but not sticky, dough.

Roll out on a floured board and use as required. If baking blind, bake at a slightly lower temperature than normal pastry, at about 180°C/350°F/Gas Mark 4.

Special occasion pastry

To cover 20 cm/8 inch pie dish

225 g/8 oz flour mix (see page 212)
¼ tsp salt
60 g/2 oz dairy-free margarine
60 g/2 oz hard white vegetable oil
60 g/2 oz icing sugar
1 large egg, beaten
½ tsp pure almond essence

Sift the flour and salt into a bowl. Add the fats and rub into a fine breadcrumb consistency. Stir in the sugar.

Stir the almond essence into the beaten egg and add sufficient to the crumbs to combine and give a soft, but not sticky, dough. Wrap in film and chill for 20 minutes.

Roll out on a floured board and use as required. If baking blind, bake on a slightly lower temperature than normal pastry, at about 180°C/350°F/Gas Mark 4.

Rice cakes

Makes 8–10 cakes

170 g/6 oz flour mix (see page 212)
115 g/4 oz ground rice
1½ tsp wheat-free baking powder (see page 214)
170 g/6 oz dairy-free margarine
170 g/6 oz caster sugar
3 eggs, beaten
pure almond essence
115 g/4 oz sultanas

Sift the flour, ground rice and baking powder together. Cream the margarine and sugar together, add the beaten eggs and almond essence a little at a time and gradually add the flour mix. Fold in the sultanas. If the mixture is too stiff, a little soya milk can be added.

Spoon into greased patty tins and bake at 190°C/375°F/Gas Mark 5 for 20 minutes.

If desired, a little water icing (120 g/4 oz icing sugar mixed with 3 tbsp warm water) can be spread over the centre of the cakes when cool.

Apple cake

For a 20 cm/8 inch cake tin

115 g/4 oz dairy-free margarine
115 g/4 oz caster sugar
few drops vanilla essence
2 large eggs, beaten
170 g/6 oz flour mix (see page 212)
1½ tsp wheat-free baking powder (see page 214)
225–280 g/8–10 oz cooking apples, peeled, cored and sliced

Topping:
115 g/4 oz flour mix (see page 212)
85 g/3 oz dairy-free margarine
85 g/3 oz soft brown sugar
2 level tsp cinnamon

Cream the fat and sugar until pale and fluffy, add the vanilla essence to the eggs and add a little at a time to the creamed mixture. Fold in the flour mixed with the baking powder. Mix to a fairly stiff dropping consistency, if necessary adding a little hot water.

Turn into a lined 20 cm/8 in loose-bottomed cake tin. Arrange the sliced apples on top of the cake mixture.

To make the topping, rub the margarine into the flour and stir in the sugar and cinnamon. Spread the topping over the apples.

Bake at 180°C/350°F/Gas Mark 4 for 1–1¼ hours or until lightly golden brown. Leave in the tin to cool.

Iced almond cakes

Makes 12–16 cakes

225 g/8 oz ground rice
170 g/6 oz caster sugar
3 eggs
pure almond essence (to taste)
120 g/4 oz icing sugar
glacé cherries
3 tbsp warm water

Grease some very small cake tins. Whisk the sugar and the eggs together for 15 minutes. Add the almond essence and ground rice. Mix well together and pour into the prepared tins.

Bake at 190°C/375°F/Gas Mark 5 for 15–20 minutes. Remove from the oven, leave to stand for 5–10 minutes and place on a wire tray.

Coat the cakes with icing made from icing sugar and water and put half a glacé cherry on top of each cake. Serve in paper cases.

Coconut fruit tarts

Makes 12–16 tarts

225 g/8 oz wheat-free shortcrust pastry (see page 220)
apricot jam
1 egg
85 g/3 oz caster sugar or fructose
115 g/4 oz desiccated coconut
dried, ready-to-eat pineapple cubes

Preheat the oven to 190°C/375°F/Gas Mark 5.
Line greased patty tins with pastry and put ½ teaspoon jam in the base of each tart. In a basin, whisk the egg well, add the sugar and mix. Add the coconut and fold in until well mixed.
Put a heaped teaspoonful of the mixture into each tart and a pineapple cube in the centre.
Bake for 20 minutes or until golden brown.

Spiced fruity rock cakes

Makes 8–10 cakes

170 g/6 oz high-fibre flour mix (see page 213)
1½ tsp wheat-free baking powder (see page 214)
½ tsp mixed spice
pinch nutmeg
pinch cinnamon
85 g/3 oz dairy-free margarine
85 g/3 oz raisins
40 g/1½ oz glacé cherries, cut into pieces
40 g/1½ oz stem ginger, chopped

1 large egg, beaten
1–2 tbsp soya milk

Line a 12-compartment patty tin with cake papers.
Sift the flour and spices into a bowl, add the margarine and rub into a breadcrumb consistency. Add the raisins, cherries and ginger. Stir to mix evenly.
Add the egg and enough milk to give a fairly stiff consistency. Divide the mixture between the paper cases.
Bake at 200°C/400°F/Gas Mark 6 for 15–20 minutes, or until cooked and lightly golden.

Chocolate cherry brownies

Makes approx 16 squares

85 g/3 oz carob dairy-free confectionery
60 g/2 oz dairy-free margarine
⅓ tsp pure vanilla essence
170 g/6 oz caster sugar
2 large eggs
85 g/3 oz flour mix plus 1 tsp wheat-free baking powder, sifted together (see pages 212, 214)
40 g/1½ oz glacé cherries, washed, dried and cut into pieces

Grease a 20 cm/8 in shallow square cake tin and line with baking parchment.
Melt the carob bar pieces in a bowl over a pan of hot water. Stir in the margarine until melted. Remove from the heat. Beat in the sugar and eggs mixed with the vanilla essence. Fold in the flour, dust the cherry pieces in flour and fold into the mixture.
Bake at 180°C/350°F/Gas Mark 4 for 25–30 minutes or until risen and firm to touch. Cut into squares.

Grandma's rice and apricot cake

For an 18 cm/7 inch cake tin

225 g/8 oz dairy-free margarine
225 g/8 oz caster sugar
170 g/6 oz flour mix with 2 tsp wheat-free baking powder
  added (see pages 212, 214)
115 g/4 oz ground rice
4 eggs
½ tsp almond essence (if not allowed, use vanilla)
tinned apricots in natural juice
little demerara sugar

Drain the juice from the apricots, dry and leave to one side.
Grease and line an 18 cm/7 in cake tin.
  Cream the margarine and sugar until pale, light and very
fluffy. Mix the flour, baking powder and ground rice together.
Add gradually in small amounts to the creamed margarine,
alternating with beaten egg. Add the almond essence and beat
to a smooth consistency. Pour into the cake tin.
  Slice the apricots into thin slices, lay gently over the top
of the mixture, sprinkle over the demerara sugar and bake
at 160°C/325°F/Gas Mark 3. Test after an hour to see if the
cake is cooked; it will take 1–1¼ hours.

Banana sultana cake

Makes 1 x 450 g/1 lb loaf

115 g/4 oz dairy-free margarine
60 g/2 oz caster sugar
2 large eggs
115 g/4 oz high-fibre flour mix and 1 tsp wheat-free baking
  powder, mixed together (see pages 213 and 214)
2 ripe bananas, mashed
60 g/2 oz walnuts, pieces or chopped (optional)

60 g/2 oz sultanas
2–3 drops vanilla essence

Line a 450 g/1 lb loaf tin with baking parchment. Cream the fat and sugar together until light and fluffy. Beat the eggs together, adding the vanilla essence.

Beat in the eggs, half at a time, adding 1 tbsp of the flour mix with the egg. Fold in the remaining flour mix and add the bananas, sultanas and walnuts. Fold in until evenly mixed.

Bake in a preheated oven at 180°C/350°F/Gas Mark 4 for 45–55 minutes or until light and springy to touch.

This cake keeps for up to three days and is suitable for freezing, whole or in individually wrapped slices.

Prune and apricot teabread

Makes 1 x 450 g/1 lb loaf

225 g/8 oz high-fibre flour mix plus 2 tsp wheat-free baking
    powder (see pages 213 and 214)
½ tsp mixed spice
½ tsp cinnamon
pinch nutmeg
140 g/5 oz dairy-free margarine
140 g/5 oz dried ready-to-eat apricots, chopped
140 g/5 oz ready-to-eat prunes, chopped
60 g/2 oz soft brown sugar
3 eggs, beaten
little soya milk (if necessary)

Place the flour, baking powder and spices in a bowl and mix. Add the margarine and rub into a breadcrumb consistency.

Stir in the sugar, apricots and prunes, add the eggs a little at a time and mix to a soft dropping consistency. Add a little soya milk if needed.

Turn into a lightly greased and lined 450 g/1 lb in loaf tin and bake for about an hour at 180°C/350°F/Gas Mark 4, or until cooked.

Pineapple and ginger cake

Makes 1 x 900 g/2 lb loaf

225 g/8 oz high-fibre flour mix (see page 213)
2 tsp wheat-free baking powder (see page 214)
1 level tsp mixed spice
60 g/2 oz soft brown sugar
115 g/4 oz dairy-free margarine
3 eggs, beaten
3–4 tbsp pineapple and ginger jam
85 g/3 oz sultanas

Beat the flour, baking powder, spice, sugar, margarine and eggs together until well mixed. Stir in the jam. Dust the sultanas with a little extra flour mix and fold them into the mixture.

Put the cake mixture in a greased and lined 900 g/2 lb loaf tin. Bake for 1–1¼ hours at 160°C/325°F/Gas Mark 3. If the cake starts to crack, reduce the oven temperature to 145°C/300°F/Gas Mark 2. Cover the top of the cake with grease-proof paper if it is browning too much.

Coconut pyramids

Makes 8–10

225 g/8 oz desiccated coconut
115 g/4 oz caster sugar
1 large egg, well beaten
½ tsp vanilla essence
little red pure food colouring (cochineal)
little cold water

Mix the coconut with the sugar, then add the beaten egg and vanilla essence and mix. If necessary, add a little cold water to make the mixture stick together. Colour with cochineal to a pale pink shade.

Take a mould or an egg-cup (rinsed well with cold water) and fill with the coconut mixture, pressing down well. Shake out the pyramids onto a greased baking sheet. Place in the refrigerator to chill for a few hours.

Remove and bake at 180°C/350°F/Gas Mark 4 for 15–20 minutes.

Victoria sponge cake

For 2 x 15–18 cm/6–7 inch sandwich tins

170 g/6 oz flour mix plus 1 tsp wheat-free baking powder
  (see pages 212, 214)
170 g/6 oz dairy-free margarine
85 g/3 oz caster sugar
3 eggs, beaten, with few drops vanilla essence
1 tbsp hot water

Preheat the oven to 190°C/375°F/Gas Mark 5. Grease and line two 15–18 cm/6–7 in sandwich tins.

Cream the margarine and sugar until pale and fluffy. Add a little egg and 1 dessertspoon of flour. Beat into the mixture and continue adding egg a little at a time, beating well.

Fold in the flour sifted with the baking powder. Add water and mix.

Divide the mixture between the two tins and bake for 20–25 minutes, or until lightly golden and firm to touch. When cold, sandwich with jam or dairy-free buttercream filling (see recipe on page 230).

Treacle scones

Makes 6–8 scones

225 g/8 oz flour mix (see page 212)
¼ tsp salt
2 tsp wheat-free baking powder (see page 214)
1 tsp mixed spice
60 g/2 oz dairy-free margarine
60 g/2 oz caster sugar
1 egg, beaten
1 tbsp black treacle
2 tbsp soya milk (if necessary)

Sift the flour into a bowl and add the salt, baking powder and mixed spice. Mix together.

Add the margarine and rub into a breadcrumb consistency. Mix in the sugar. Add the treacle to the beaten egg and mix well to combine. Pour into the flour and mix into a soft, but not sticky, dough, adding a little soya milk if necessary.

Roll out the dough on a floured board and cut into 4 cm/1½ in scones.

Bake in the oven at 200°C/400°F/Gas Mark 6 for 10–12 minutes, or until cooked.

Cinnamon shortbread

Makes 8–10 pieces

115 g/4 oz flour mix plus 1 tsp wheat-free baking powder
   (see pages 212, 214)
85 g/3 oz dairy-free margarine
115 g/4 oz caster sugar
2 egg yolks
2 level tsp cinnamon
little demerara sugar and cinnamon

Rub the margarine into the flour to a breadcrumb consistency. Stir in the sugar and cinnamon and add the egg yolks. It should be a fairly stiff dough. If necessary, add a little soya milk.

Roll out on a floured board to thickness of about 1 cm/½ in. Brush the top with soya milk and sprinkle with a mixture of demerara sugar and cinnamon.

Bake at 180°C/350°F/Gas Mark 4 for 15–20 minutes, or until lightly golden.

Pear and carob cake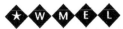

115 g/4 oz dairy-free margarine
140 g/5 oz rice flour
30 g/1 oz carob flour
85 g/3 oz soya flour
115 g/4 oz brown sugar
2 pears, stewed, cooled and liquidized
1–2 tbsp soya milk
1 level tsp sodium bicarbonate in 2 tsp water

Filling:
60 g/2 oz dairy-free margarine
85 g/3 oz icing sugar

Preheat the oven to 180°C/350°F/Gas Mark 4.

Rub the margarine into the flours, then add the sugar. Mix thoroughly. Make a well in the centre and slowly stir in the pears and milk substitute until all the flour has been taken up; the mixture should be slightly sloppy. Add the bicarbonate of soda and water. Beat the mixture hard until it becomes smooth and fluffy. This is important: if the beating does not reach this stage the cake will be flat and unpalatable.

Turn immediately into two 18 cm/7 in greased cake tins. Bake for 25–30 minutes.

For the filling, cream the margarine, add sugar gradually and beat together.

When the cake is cool, sandwich the two halves together with the filling.

Rice Krispie cakes

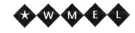

Makes 20–24 cakes

2 tbsp honey or golden syrup
30 g/1 oz brown sugar
at least 30 g/1 oz Rice Krispies

Heat the honey and sugar until the sugar dissolves. Stir in enough Rice Krispies to absorb the honey. Spoon into paper cases and leave to cool and harden.

Alternatives: chopped dates or 2 tsp carob flour may be added.

Iced gingernuts

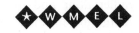

Makes 12–16

30 g/1 oz dairy-free margarine
30 g/1 oz soft brown sugar
60 g/2 oz golden syrup
60 g/2 oz soya flour
30 g/1 oz rice flour
1 tsp wheat-free baking powder (see page 214)
½ tsp cream of tartar
½ tsp ground ginger
120 g/4 oz icing sugar
3 tbsp warm water

Preheat the oven to 180°C/350°F/Gas Mark 4.
    Melt the margarine in a pan on low heat and stir in the golden syrup and sugar. Sift together the dry ingredients and then re-sift them into the pan. Stir to a firm paste. Take small spoonfuls and roll in the hands until smooth (walnut size), then flatten on a greased baking tray. Bake for 15–17 minutes.
    Leave to cool, then mix together the sugar and water to make the water icing and decorate.

Date and millet squares

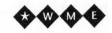

Makes 16 squares

225 g/8 oz dates, chopped
115 ml/4 fl oz apple juice
115 g/4 oz dairy-free margarine
170 g/6 oz soft brown sugar
115 g/4 oz rice or millet flour
170 g/6 oz millet flakes

Preheat the oven to 180°C/350°F/Gas Mark 4.

Put the dates in a pan, pour in the apple juice and cook over a gentle heat until the mixture is soft and pulpy (about 5 minutes). Chop the margarine into small pieces. Place the sugar, rice or millet flour and millet flakes in a bowl, add the chopped margarine and mix until all the ingredients are combined.

Grease an 18 x 23 cm/7 x 9 in baking tin. Divide the millet mixture in half. Press half the mixture firmly into the bottom of the tin and spread the date mixture over the top. Cover with the remaining millet mixture and press down firmly.

Bake for 35–40 minutes. Allow to cool in the tin. Cut into squares when cold.

Eggless fruit cake

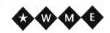

For a 20 cm/8 in diameter cake tin

450 ml/¾ pint water
115 g/4 oz currants
115 g/4 oz raisins
225 g/8 oz dairy-free margarine
170 g/6 oz demerara sugar
115 g/4 oz millet flour
115 g/4 oz rice flour
1 tbsp wheat-free baking powder (see page 214)
1 tsp bicarbonate of soda
1 tsp mixed spice

Preheat the oven to 190°C/375°F/Gas Mark 5.

Put the water, currants, raisins, margarine and sugar in a pan and bring to the boil. Simmer for 5 minutes. Leave to cool.

Sift the millet flour, rice flour, baking powder, bicarbonate of soda and mixed spice together three times. When the ingredients in the pan are quite cold mix them with the flour mixture until thoroughly combined.

Grease a loose-bottomed 20 cm/8 in cake tin with margarine. Fill with the mixture and bake for 2 hours. Leave the cake to cool in the tin for a few minutes before turning it onto a wire tray.

Recipes using an all-purpose flour mix

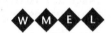

500 g/18 oz brown rice flour
1500 g/53 oz white rice flour
500 g/18 oz tapioca starch
500 g/18 oz farina (potato starch)

This is an excellent all-purpose mix, which can also be used to bake the items listed in previous pages. It is light for cakes, pastry and, especially, steamed puddings. The brown rice flour adds a good binding consistency, but if a heavier flour is needed, for example in rich fruit cakes, you can add some xanthan gum. This is readily available from health-food shops. Take care to check whether it is derived from corn or soya. Gluten-free bread will not rise without xanthan-gum. For those with multiple intolerances, flat breads are easy to make and can be very tasty. They can be ground into breadcrumbs and frozen for use in other recipes. All alternative flours should be kept in a freezer. This will extend shelf-life and prevent mustiness.

Potato bread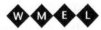

225 g/8 oz raw potatoes, peeled and grated
225 g/8 oz cooked potato, cooled and mashed
225 g/8 oz all-purpose flour mix (see page 233)
½ tsp salt
a pinch celery salt
a pinch pure white pepper
60 g/2 oz dairy-free margarine, melted

Mix the raw and mashed potatoes together, then stir in the flour, salt, celery salt, pepper and melted margarine. Mix well to just combine but do not over handle. Divide the dough into two pieces, press out each piece into a flat round and place on two greased baking sheets. Bake in the oven at 150°C/300°F/Gas mark 2 for 40 minutes. Cut into pieces and serve hot.

Chapattis

225 g/8 oz all-purpose flour mix (see page 233)
1 tsp xanthan gum
a large pinch salt
30 g/1 oz pure sunflower margarine
150 ml/5 fl oz water
1 tbsp sunflower oil

Mix the flour, xanthan gum and salt in a bowl, rub in the margarine until the mixture is a fine breadcrumb consistency. Mix in the water to form a stiff dough. Knead on a lightly floured board for 10 minutes. Cover the dough on the board and leave to rest for 30 minutes.

Divide the dough into 8 pieces and roll out each piece into a 12 cm/5 in circle.

Heat the oil in a pan and fry each chapatti for 3 minutes, turning frequently. Drain on kitchen paper and serve warm.

Baking powder bread

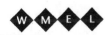

450 g/1 lb all-purpose flour mix (see page 233)
2 tsp xanthan gum
1 tbsp baking powder
pinch of salt
150 ml/¼ pint water mixed with 150ml/¼ pint rice
   or soya milk

Preheat the oven to 220°C/425°F/Gas Mark 7. Sift the flour, xanthan gum, salt and baking powder into a bowl. Add the milk and water mix and combine to a firm dough, but do not knead. Divide into two pieces and shape to fit into two 450 g/1 lb greased loaf tins. Brush the top with milk, bake for 25 minutes.

Eat as soon as possible as this bread does not keep. Any left over can be put into a grinder and made into bread crumbs to keep in the freezer ready for other recipes that call for breadcrumbs.

When the top is brushed with milk/water, it can be sprinkled with poppy seeds, which give extra flavour.

Yoghurt bread

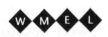

340 g/12 oz all-purpose flour mix (see page 233)
115 g/4 oz rice bran ground to a fine crumb
2 tsp xanthan gum
4 tsp wheat-free baking powder (see page 214)
2 tsp light, soft brown sugar
1 tsp salt
150 ml/¼ pint live soya yoghurt
150 ml/¼ pint water

Preheat the oven to 220°C/425°F/Gas Mark 7.

Mix the flour, baking powder, xanthan gum, sugar and salt together in a bowl.

Add the yoghurt and enough water to make a soft dough. Knead well and shape to fit a greased 450 g/1 lb loaf tin. Bake for 45 minutes and cool on a wire rack.

Quickie biscuits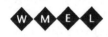

Makes 18

115 g/4 oz dairy-free margarine
60 g/2 oz caster sugar
140 g/5 oz all-purpose flour mix (see page 233)
1½ tsp wheat-free baking powder (see page 214)

Preheat the oven to 180°C/350°F/Gas Mark 4. Cream the margarine and sugar until light and fluffy. Gradually stir in the flour mixed with the baking powder. Using your hands, form a soft dough. Roll into small balls and place wide apart on a greased baking tray. Dip a fork in cold water to flatten and mark across the top of the biscuits.

Bake for 12–15 minutes on until pale golden. Cool for 5 minutes before removing biscuits to a cooling rack.

Sweet potato and pineapple cake

450 g/1 lb sweet potato peeled and cut into chunks
115 g/4 oz dairy-free margarine
4 tbsp fresh pineapple juice
170 g/6 oz soft light brown sugar
3 medium eggs, separated
170 g/6 oz all-purpose flour mix (see page 233)
2 level tsp wheat-free baking powder (see page 214)
1 tsp cinnamon

Preheat oven to 180°C/350°F/Gas Mark 4. Put the potato chunks into a pan of lightly salted boiling water and cook for 10 minutes or until tender. Drain the potatoes, add the margarine and mash really well. Leave to cool.

Put the pineapple juice into a bowl with the sugar and whisk well. Add the egg yolks and beat well to a smooth mixture. Pour in the sweet potato mixture and stir to combine.

Whisk the egg whites until they form stiff peaks. Fold 1 tbsp of egg white into the sweet potato mix to loosen it, then continue to add egg white 1 tbsp at a time until all is combined.

Mix the baking powder and cinnamon into the flour and then fold into the mixture. Gently pour into a 1½ kg/3 lb loaf tin, greased and lined with baking parchment, and bake for approx 1 hour or until a knife inserted in the cake comes out clean. Check the top for over browning, and if necessary cover with tin foil.

Leave the cake in the tin until just warm. Serve warm as a pudding with a slice of pineapple and yoghurt, or serve cold as a teabread.

Date loaf

225 g/8 oz chopped dates
150 ml/5 fl oz rice or soya milk
3½ tbsp clear honey or rice syrup
1 egg
225 g/8 oz all-purpose flour mix (see page 233)
1 tsp xanthan gum
2 ½ tsp wheat-free baking powder (see page 214)
¼ tsp nutmeg
little dairy-free margarine

Preheat oven to 180°C/350°F/Gas Mark 4. Simmer the dates in the milk for about 10 minutes, until soft. Sift together the flour, xanthan gum, baking powder and nutmeg. Remove the dates from the heat, beat 3 tablespoons of honey (or rice syrup), and the egg into the mixture. Transfer the mixture to a blender and purée. Return the mixture to a clean bowl and fold in the flour mix.

Turn the mixture into a prepared 900 g/2 lb loaf tin and bake for about 1 hour or until firm and lightly browned.

Gooey flapjacks

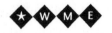

140 g/5 oz dairy-free margarine
115 g/4 oz apricot jam
2 heaped tbsp golden syrup
340 g/12 oz rice and millet flakes, mixed and very lightly
    toasted
1 level tsp cinnamon
½ tsp wheat-free baking powder (see page 214)
2 medium-sized ripe bananas

Preheat oven to 180°C. Melt together the margarine, jam and syrup in a large saucepan over a low heat and stir in the mixed flakes, cinnamon, baking powder and a pinch of salt until well combined.

Peel and mash the bananas and add to the mixture, combining thoroughly.

Pour the mixture into a greased Swiss roll tin, bake for about 20 minutes or until the edges are turning golden. The mixture will be fairly firm.

Transfer the tin to a wire rack, cut into bars while still hot but do not remove from tin until completely cold.

Moreish carrot cake

170 g/6 oz muscovado sugar
170 ml/6 fl oz sunflower oil
3 large eggs, beaten
140 g/5 oz grated carrot
115 g/4 oz sultanas
170 g/6 oz all-purpose flour mix (see page 233)
2 level tsp of wheat-free baking powder (see page 214)
1 tsp bicarbonate of soda
1 tsp groung cinnamon
½ tsp grated nutmeg
pinch wheat-free mixed spice
Preheat the oven to 180°C/350°F/Gas Mark 4. Put the

sugar and oil in a large mixing bowl, add the eggs and lightly mix with a wooden spoon, stir in the carrots and the sultanas.

Sift together flour, baking powder, bicarbonate of soda and spices into the mixing bowl and lightly mix all the ingredients together.

Pour the mixture into a greased and lined cake tin and bake for about 40 minutes or until it is springy to touch.

For a topping, mix a little liquidized fresh pineapple with some plain toffutti and spread thinly over the cake when cold.

Caribbean cakes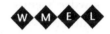

Makes 10

225 g/8 oz all-purpose flour mix (see page 233)
½ tsp salt
3 tsp wheat-free baking powder (see page 214)
60 g/2 oz dairy-free margarine
2–3 tbsp grated coconut (if using desiccated coconut moisten
   with 1 tbsp of water)
sunflower oil for frying

Sieve the flour mix with the salt and the baking powder in a large bowl. Rub in the margarine until coarse breadcrumbs form. Add the grated coconut and then gradually mix in 150 ml/¼ pint water (a little more may be necessary to make a soft but firm dough). With floured hands, roll the dough into 10 balls, golf ball size, flattening each one a little.

Heat the oil in a deep frying pan and fry the cakes for 5 minutes each side over a moderate heat.

Vanilla sponge loaf

140 g/5 fl oz sunflower oil (preferably 'buttery' variety)
4 large eggs

2 tbsp caster sugar, or 2 tbsp apricot jam
225 g/8 oz all-purpose flour mix (see page 233)
2 tsp wheat-free baking powder (see page 214)
1½ tsp pure vanilla essence

Preheat the oven to 180°C/350°F/Gas Mark 4.

Warm a glass bowl and whisk together the eggs, vanilla and choice of sweetening until the mixture is thick (about 6–8 minutes), using an electric whisk.

Slowly add the buttery oil, whisking all the time on the lowest speed. The mixture should now be very thick.

In a separate bowl, sift together the flour and baking powder. Gently fold the flour into the egg mixture until it is combined.

Gently spoon into a greased, lined 900 g/2 lb loaf tin. Bake for about 50 minutes or until a knife inserted in the loaf comes out clean.

Slimmers cake with fruit sauce

Cake:
2 eggs
60 g/2 oz caster sugar
60 g/2 oz all-purpose flour mix (see page 233)
1 tsp cinnamon

Sauce:
2 tbsp clear honey
300 ml/½ pint fresh pineapple juice
2 tbsp rum (if allowed)

Preheat the oven to 180°C/350°F/Gas Mark 4.

In a large mixing bowl, whisk the eggs and sugar with an electric whisk until the mixture leaves a trail on the surface when whisk is lifted (about 5–6 minutes).

Sift over the flour and cinnamon and then very gently fold in, using a metal spoon.

Pour the mixture into a 20 cm/8 in cake tin greased and lined with baking parchment. Bake for 15–20 minutes until lightly golden and spongy to the touch. Leave for 10 minutes before transferring to a wire cooling rack.

To make the sauce, boil all the sauce ingredients together until reduced to a syrup. Cut cake into wedges, dust with icing sugar and serve drizzled with the sauce.

Butternut squash and spiced loaf

170 g/6 oz dairy-free margarine
170 g/6 oz clear honey
1 large egg, beaten
280 g/10 oz peeled butternut squash, coarsely grated
115 g/4 oz light muscovado sugar
340 g/12 oz all-purpose flour mix (see page 233)
3 heaped tsp wheat-free baking powder (see page 214)
1 dessertspoon ground ginger
1 tsp gluten-free mixed spice

Preheat the oven to 180°C/350°F/Gas Mark 4.

Mix the margarine, honey and egg and stir in the butternut squash.

Mix in the sugar, flour, spice and ginger.

Pour the mixture into a 1 kg/2 lb loaf tin, greased and lined with baking parchment.

Bake for about 1 hour on until risen and golden. Leave to cool slightly before transferring to a cooling rack.

Can be served with dairy-free spread or apricot or mango and ginger jam.

Blackberry and apple cake

170 g/6 oz dairy-free margarine
170 g/6 oz caster sugar
3 large eggs
170 g/6 oz all-purpose flour mix (see page 233)

2 level tsp of wheat-free baking powder (see page 214)
225 g/8 oz blackberries
2 Golden Delicious apples, peeled, cored and diced

Preheat the oven to 180°C/350°F/Gas Mark 4.

Cream the butter and sugar together until light and fluffy, beat in the eggs, one at a time. Fold in the flour mixed with the baking powder. Spoon ¾ of the mixture into a greased and lined 23 cm/9 in cake tin, with spring release. Spread the fruit over the mixture.

Drop spoonfuls of the remaining mixture in an irregular pattern over the top of the fruit.

Bake for about 1 hour or until risen and golden. Cool in the tin.

Beverages

Honey cold-soother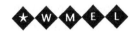

honey
1 clove
¼ tsp cinnamon
few grains nutmeg

Pour a mug of water into a pan, add a large spoonful of honey, the clove, cinnamon and nutmeg and bring to the boil, stirring continuously. Strain and cool for at least a few minutes before drinking.

Peppermint bracer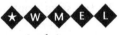

1–2 drops pure peppermint oil (use very sparingly)
few grains caster sugar
1–2 tbsp apple juice

Put the peppermint oil and sugar into a jug and pour on a mugful of hot water just off the boil. Stir in the apple juice. Leave to cool to a drinkable heat.

Mango and ginger warmer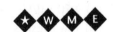

½ mango, liquidized
300 ml/½ pint soya milk
pinch ground ginger
little honey if required

Gently heat the soya milk and stir in the ginger. When the milk is at the required heat, briskly stir in the liquidized mango.

Spicy cinnamon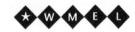

300 ml/½ pint soya milk
generous pinch cinnamon
small pinch nutmeg
1 tbsp black treacle

Pour the milk into a saucepan, add the cinnamon, a few grains of nutmeg and the black treacle. Heat gently to just below boiling, stirring continuously.

Banana milkshake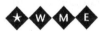

1 ripe banana, cut into slices
1 mug or cup soya milk or rice milk, chilled
¼ tsp soya yoghurt

Place all the ingredients in a liquidizer, process and chill.

Other fruit milkshakes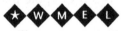

Take ¾ tumbler of chilled soya milk or rice milk, some crushed ice and make your choice of milkshake by adding one of the following:

(a) 150 ml/¼ pint raspberry purée
(b) few fresh strawberries
(c) few slices pineapple
(d) heaped tbsp blackcurrants
(e) rosehip syrup – follow instructions on bottle

Put the milk and fruit in a liquidizer, process until smooth, pour into a jug and add the crushed ice.

Fruit purée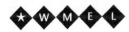

If you prefer not to use milk, you can blend or liquidize the following:

1 pear, peeled, cored and chopped
2 or 3 apricots, depending on size, with crushed ice

Alternatively, try the 100 per cent pure green/white grape juice, now available from supermarkets, chilled with crushed ice and a drop of peppermint.

Vegetable drinks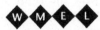

Most of us have our own favourite tomato juice recipes. Try adding carrot juice to yours with a pinch of salt. Possible new favourites include celery and cucumber with crushed ice.

Children's recipes

Potato fingers

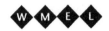

Serves 1 adult, or 2 children

30 g/1 oz all-purpose flour mix (see page 233)
225 g/8 oz mashed potato
salt and pepper
little rice or soya milk or a little beaten egg

Mix the flour with the mashed potato and season to taste.
If necessary, bind with a little beaten egg or suitable milk.
Shape into fingers, glaze with egg or milk, bake in a hot oven
for about 10 minutes until lightly brown and crisp

Potato floddies

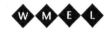

Makes 1

2 potatoes scrubbed
a little wheat- and corn-free flour
salt and pepper
a little sunflower oil

Coarsely grate the potatoes over a bowl and add sufficient
flour to form a batter. Season with salt and pepper. Put a
little oil in a non-stick pan and heat until quite hot. Drop
the mixture into it. When brown underneath, turn and brown
the other side.

Serve with a little jam spread over or some stewed fruit
(all juice drained) for a sweet dish.

Alternatively this can be spread with scrambled egg or
another savoury topping.

Chicken burgers

Serves 6

450 g/1 lb minced chicken
170 g/6 oz minced turkey
115 g/4 oz lean bacon, finely chopped
2 tbsp fresh chives, chopped
1 tbsp fresh lemon thyme, chopped
little beaten egg, if necessary
little wheat-free flour mix (see page 212)

Place the first five ingredients in a food processor, pulse until mixture is combined. If necessary add a very small amount of beaten egg and pulse again. Remove the mixture to a floured board. With floured hands shape into balls and then flatten. Dust with the flour and fry in sunflower oil.

Sausage and bean loaf

450 g/1 lb fresh minced chicken
170 g/6 oz fresh minced turkey plus 115 g/4 oz minced lean
  bacon
1 tbsp fresh parsley and thyme, finely chopped
1 tbsp tomato purée
salt and freshly ground black pepper

Stuffing:
Can of baked beans, wheat-free
60 g/2 oz cooked rice
2 tbsp tomato purée

Preheat the oven to 190°C/375°F/Gas Mark 5.

Mix the loaf ingredients together in a bowl. Press half of this mixture into a lightly greased 900 g/2 lb loaf tin.

Mix the stuffing ingredients together and spread over the meat mixture in the tin.

Add the remaining meat mixture, smooth the top and press down firmly with a flat spatula.

Bake for about 1 hour, or until cooked.

This can be frozen in slices and used for packed lunches or served with salad, warm or cold.

Chicken nuggets

Serves 2–3 children

1 chicken breast, boned and skinned
60 g/2 oz wheat-free breadcrumbs or ground rice
¼ tsp paprika pepper
1½ tbsp wheat-free flour mix (see page 212)
1 egg, beaten (or white of 1 egg)
salt and pepper
oil for frying

Flatten the chicken breast to required thickness and cut into shapes. Mix the breadcrumbs with the seasonings.

Toss the chicken in the flour, dip in the beaten egg and then coat in the breadcrumbs. Fry until golden.

Oven baked crumbed fish

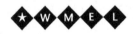

30 g/1 oz suitable breadcrumbs
¼ tsp dried oregano, or 1 tbsp fresh parsley, chopped
pinch paprika pepper
100 ml/4 fl oz rice or soya milk
1 piece of cod fillet (cod loin, although expensive, does cut
    into fingers very well, is meaty and substantial)
little melted dairy-free margarine

Preheat the oven to 220°C/425°F/Gas Mark 7. Grease an

ovenproof dish, combine the breadcrumbs, chopped herb and paprika on a plate. Put the milk in a bowl, add a pinch of salt and stir well.

Cut the fish into finger-sizes, then dip first in milk and then in crumb mixture. Arrange in a prepared dish in single layer. Drizzle a little melted butter over the fish.

Bake for 10–15 minutes or until fish flakes easily with a fork.

Potato carrot cake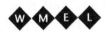

mashed potato
carrot, diced and cooked
sunflower oil

Well-seasoned mashed potato combined with cooked carrot makes a wholesome and savoury-tasting pancake.

Using electric beaters, whip some mashed potatoes to a loose creamy consistency (no need to add milk or fat if you use electric beaters). Season well with salt and pepper. Add some diced cooked carrot.

Pan fried in a little sunflower oil, it develops a delicious crisp crust but it can be baked to a golden brown in the oven if preferred.

Fruity jellies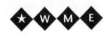

225 g/8 oz no-need-to-soak apricots
300 ml/½ pint suitable fruit juice (such as white grape or pear juice)
3 tsp apricot jam
1 tbsp powdered gelatine (vegetable gelatine leaves are best for correct measurement)
4 tbsp boiling water

Put the apricots in a saucepan and pour in the fruit juice. Bring to the boil, cover and simmer for 15–20 minutes until plump and soft. Leave to cool for 10 minutes.

Transfer the mixture to a blender and process until smooth, add the jam and process again until smooth.

Pour the mixture into a measuring jug and make up to 1 pint with cold water.

Dissolve the gelatine in the boiling water and stir into the apricot mixture. Pour the mixture into 4 individual moulds, 150 ml/5 fl oz size. Leave to chill and set.

For a red jelly, use pears instead of apricots. As pears have a higher water content than apricots, add a little less cold water at first until you judge the set. Flavour with black cherry jam and add 2–3 drops of pure vegetable colouring (nut free).

For a green jelly, use pears instead of apricots and add a little green pure vegetable colouring such as peppermint colouring. (Check it is nut free.)

Chocolate custard

Serves 4

2 egg yolks
225 ml/8 fl oz rice or soya milk
60 g/2 oz carob bar (wheat- and dairy-free)
30 g/1 oz sugar

Heat the milk until very hot, add the carob bar and stir until melted.

Beat the egg yolks and sugar together until pale and creamy.

Slowly pour the milk onto the egg mixture, stirring all the time, and blend well.

Return the mixture to the pan and heat over a low to medium heat, still stirring constantly, until the sauce thickens.

To make a mousse-type treat thicken with a little cornflour

(make sure it is wheat-free) and pour into a mould. Leave to set.

A special treat

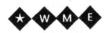

Serves 1

½ mango
1 banana
1–2 kiwi fruits, or 1 pear
live soya yoghurt
carob bar (wheat- and dairy-free)

Cut the mango into pieces and liquidize. Add to the yoghurt and combine well.

Mash the banana and finely chop the kiwi fruits (or pear).

Put a little banana in the bottom of a tallish glass, put in a layer of the yoghurt mix, add a layer of the chopped kiwi (or pear) then another layer of the yoghurt mix each time. Chill.

Just before serving, grate a little of the carob bar over the top.

Nursery apple pudding

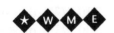

Serves 6–8

450 g/1 lb Golden Delicious apples, peeled cored and chopped
1 pineapple jelly (check ingredients)

Poach the fruit in 600 ml/1 pint of water, cooking until very soft and mushy. Remove from heat (can be liquidized if desired) Stir in the jelly cubes while apple is still hot, and keep stirring until dissolved completely.

Pour into mould and leave to set.

Christmas

Almost a punch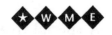

Serves 3

600 ml/1 pint pure red grape juice
little demerara sugar to taste
2 cloves and 2 good pinches cinnamon
260 ml/½ pint water or mango juice

Put all the ingredients in a pan, gently warm through to medium heat, strain and serve in warmed glasses.

Festive salmon mousse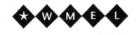

Serves 4

150 ml/¼ pint aspic jelly
few mint leaves
few slices cucumber
30 g/1 oz dairy-free margarine
30 g/1 oz gram flour (or any suitable flour used for thickening)
300 ml/½ pint soya milk
220 g/7¾ oz tin pink salmon
100 g/3½ oz soya cream
salt and pepper
15 g/½ oz vegetable gelatine

Make up the aspic jelly as directed. Rinse a round 15 cm/ 6 in cake tin with cold water, pour half the aspic jelly into the base and leave it in a cool place to set.

Wash and dry the mint leaves. Dip the mint leaves and cucumber in the aspic jelly and arrange them decoratively on the set jelly in the tin. Leave to set. Then pour on the remaining aspic and leave to set.

Melt the margarine in a pan, stir in the flour for 2 minutes, then remove from the heat. Stir in the milk, return to the heat and bring to the boil, stirring constantly. Simmer for 2 minutes.

Drain the salmon and remove any skin and bones. Stir the salmon and cream into the sauce and season to taste.

Dissolve the gelatine in 2 tbsp cold water and stir into the salmon mixture. Allow to cool. Pour salmon mixture into tin and allow to set in refrigerator.

When ready to serve, dip the tin in hot water for a few seconds, turn onto a plate and garnish.

Stuffed turkey breast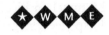

Serves 6–8

breast of turkey, 1½–2½ kg/3½–5 lb in weight
280 g/10 oz unsmoked lean bacon
2 leeks, washed and cut into fine rings
2–3 level tsp oregano
sunflower oil

Open out the breast of turkey, wipe clean and trim off any odd pieces of skin. Beat any extra-thick parts with a rolling pin until the meat is a fairly even thickness all over.

Trim the bacon and lay rashers across the turkey to line the inside. Scatter rings of leeks all over and sprinkle the oregano over the leeks. Roll up the breast lengthways and tie at intervals with string.

Place the turkey on a sheet of baking foil and brush well with oil. Fold the foil over to loosely enclose it. Bake for approximately 20 mins/lb plus an extra 20 minutes at 190°C/375°F/Gas Mark 5, reducing to 180°C/340°F/Gas Mark 4 after the first hour, brushing at intervals. Open up the foil for the last 30 minutes and allow the turkey to brown.

Pork fillet with spiced peaches and cream

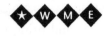

Serves 4

450 g/1 lb pork fillet, trimmed and prepared
salt and freshly ground black pepper
2 or 3 large peaches (450 g/1 lb in weight approx)
225–280 ml/8–10 fl oz white grape juice
60 g/2 oz caster sugar
2 whole cloves garlic
2 whole allspice
25 mm/1 in piece cinnamon stick
1 tsp rice vinegar
little soya cream

Season the pork fillet and loosely wrap it in lightly greased oven foil. Place in a roasting tin and cook for 30–40 minutes or until the juices run clear and meat is tender, at 180°C/350°F/Gas Mark 4.

Meanwhile, plunge the peaches into boiling water and skin them. Slice each peach in half and then each half into three. Put the grape juice, sugar, garlic, spices and vinegar in a saucepan and bring to the boil. Simmer for 10 minutes, then spoon the peach slices into the syrup and simmer for a further 5–6 minutes. Remove the peaches and keep warm. Boil the syrup to reduce by about a third to a half.

Remove from the heat, discard the garlic and spices and add the juices from the pork to the remaining syrup. Swirl in some soya cream. Spoon a little of the spiced cream syrup onto each plate and add slices of pork fillet with peach slices arranged between.

The Christmas ham

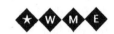

Serves 4–6

1–1½ kg/2–3 lb joint of gammon
2 tbsp clear honey

1 large mango, stone removed and flesh chopped
little pineapple juice
pinch of either allspice or cinnamon or cloves (optional)

The day before cooking, rinse the gammon in cold water, put in a large bowl, cover with cold water and leave overnight.

Next day, remove from the bowl and rinse with fresh clean water. Put the joint in a saucepan, cover with cold water, bring to the boil and boil for 2 minutes. Drain and rinse with cold water again; this should remove all excess salt.

Dry the gammon and place it on a large sheet of foil. Spread a thin covering of honey over the surface of the gammon and bake at 160°C/325°F/Gas Mark 3 for half the required cooking time (total cooking time approx 20 mins/lb plus an extra 20 minutes), basting in the juices at intervals. Remove from the oven, open the foil and add the chopped mango to the gammon. Pour over the pineapple juice, sprinkle over the pinch of spice if using, re-wrap the joint and return it to oven, basting frequently.

Thirty minutes before the end of the cooking time, open the foil and allow the gammon to become lightly golden. Do not let the mango over-brown.

Braised venison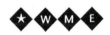

115–170 g/4–6 oz lean venison per person
lean bacon
chestnut mushrooms, sliced
a little wheat- and corn-free flour
a little oil
good-quality stock (see page 190)
sprigs parsley
1 sprig thyme
small sprig rosemary

Heat the oil in a pan on top of stove. Cube the venison and

roll in the seasoned flour. Lightly brown off in the hot oil, and add the bacon for the last 2 minutes.

Transfer the meat, bacon and stock to an ovenproof dish with lid, and add the mushrooms, parsley, thyme and rosemary.

Transfer to the oven set at 140°C/275°F/Gas Mark 1 and cook slowly and gently for about 2–3 hours.

Thicken liquid if required with flour or arrowroot.

Serve with crushed potatoes and steamed vegetables.

Celery and tomato stuffing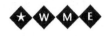

Serves 2–3

170 g/6 oz cooked white rice
60 g/2 oz celery, chopped finely
2 tomatoes, skinned, seeded and chopped
2 tsp mixed herbs
salt and pepper to taste
1 egg white, beaten, or 1–2 tbsp dairy-free margarine, melted

Combine all the ingredients except the last, adding the egg white or melted margarine to bring the mixture together.

Leek, mushroom and apple stuffing

Serves 2

115 g/4 oz cooked brown rice
60 g/2 oz leeks, cut into fine rings
60 g/2 oz chestnut or button mushrooms, chopped
60 g/2 oz stewed apple
salt and pepper
1 egg white, beaten

Combine the first four ingredients in a bowl, season to taste, add the egg white and mix well. If the mixture is too stiff, add a spoonful of hot water.

A pudding to enjoy

Serves 6–8

115 g/4 oz flour mix (see page 212)
115 g/4 oz wheat-free soda breadcrumbs (see page 214)
225 g/8 oz soft dark brown sugar
pinch salt
pinch nutmeg
225 ml/8 fl oz sunflower oil (preferably 'buttery' variety)
225 g/8 oz currants
225 g/8 oz raisins
225 g/8 oz sultanas
2 large eggs
150 ml/¼ pint soya milk
60 g/2 oz toasted pine nuts
little rum or brandy to taste (optional)

Mix all the ingredients together except the rum or brandy (if using), then stir in the liquor and leave to stand overnight.

Mix again and spoon into a 1.5 litre/3½ pint basin. Cover with double thickness of grease-proof paper and then tin foil. Steam for at least 6–8 hours.

The longer you steam this pudding, the tastier it will be.

Christmas cake

For a 18–20 cm/7–8 in cake tin

225 g/8 oz high-fibre flour mix, mixed with 60 g/2 oz wheat-free baking powder (see pages 213, 214)
½ tsp natural pectin or 2 tsp xanthan gum
1 tsp mixed spice

pinch cinnamon
115 g/4 oz soft dark brown sugar
1 tbsp black treacle
340 g/12 oz mixed currants, sultanas, raisins
60 g/2 oz glacé cherries, washed and chopped
few drops almond essence
2 large eggs, beaten
115 ml/4 fl oz sunflower oil (preferably 'buttery' variety)
115 ml/4 fl oz soya milk

Sift the flour and baking powder into a bowl, then stir in the powdered pectin, spices, sugar, dried fruit and cherries.

Mix together the beaten eggs, treacle, oil, milk and almond essence. Add to the dry ingredients and mix to an even dropping consistency.

Bake in greased and lined 18–20 cm/7–8 in cake tin at 160°C/325°F/Gas Mark 3 for 1½–1¾ hours, or until cooked.

Eggless festive cake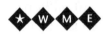

For a 20 cm/8 in cake tin

225 g/8 oz flour mix and 2 tsp wheat- and corn-free baking
   powder (see pages 212, 214), sifted together
1 tsp mixed spice
pinch nutmeg
170 g/6 oz mixed currants, sultanas, raisins
60 g/2 oz glacé cherries, washed and chopped
200 ml/7 fl oz soya milk
340 g/12 oz golden syrup
225 g/8 oz dairy-free margarine, melted
few drops vanilla essence
½ tsp natural pectin or 2 tsp xanthan gum

Stir the golden syrup into melted margarine and add the vanilla essence. Mix together all the dry ingredients, and then add the milk, margarine and syrup mixture.

Spoon into greased and lined 20 cm/8 in cake tin and bake at 150°C/300°F/Gas Mark 2 for 1–1½ hours, or until cooked.

When cool, double wrap the cake (one layer of grease-proof and one layer of foil), place it in an airtight container and leave for at least a week.

Mincemeat of a kind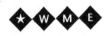

115 g/4 oz sultanas
115 g/4 oz raisins
85 g/3 oz glacé cherries, washed free of sugar
60 g/2 oz dried, ready-to-eat apricots
85 g/3 oz eating apple, grated
2 tbsp white grape juice
1 tsp clear honey
1 tsp cinnamon
1 tsp allspice
pinch nutmeg
2 tbsp brandy or rum (optional, but it does help to preserve)
1 tbsp toasted pine nuts

Mince or finely chop the fruits and put into a bowl. Put the grape juice, honey, spices and brandy/rum (if using) into a small pan. Bring to the boil and simmer for 2 minutes. Remove from the heat.

Pour into a clean jug to cool quickly. When just warm, pour over the fruits and mix thoroughly, but do not beat. Adjust the quantity of liquid at this stage. Finally, fold in the pine nuts.

Spoon into clean, sterile jars, with tight-fitting lids. Stored in the refrigerator, this mincemeat will keep for 3–4 weeks.

Mincemeat pie filling

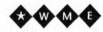

170 g/6 oz chopped apples and pears
255 g/9 oz mixed dried fruit
30 g/1 oz glacé cherries, chopped
few drops vanilla essence
85 g/3 oz soft brown sugar (molasses is good)
1 tsp cinnamon
good pinch of nutmeg
2 tbsp white grape or pineapple juice
85 ml/3 fl oz brandy (omit for exclusion diet)

Put all the ingredients in a pan and simmer over a low heat
for 35–40 minutes, stirring frequently. Allow to cool, pack
into clean, sterile jars, seal and store in the refrigerator.

Appendix A

Foods containing cow's milk and cow's milk products

Milk is used in a variety of manufactured products. Check all labels on bought foods and if the following items are included do not use that product: milk, butter, margarine, cream, cheese, yoghurt, skimmed milk powder, non-fat milk solids, caseinates, whey, lactalbumin, lactose.

The foods listed below are likely to contain milk and/or milk products, so always check the list of ingredients.

biscuits
bread, bread mixes
breakfast cereals
cakes, cake mixes
gravy mixes
malted milk drinks, e.g. Horlicks, Ovaltine, Bournvita
puddings and mixes, e.g. ice-cream, instant whips, custards
ready meals – fish, meat, rice and pasta dishes
sauces, cream soups
sausages
sweets, e.g. milk chocolate, fudge, toffee
vegetables canned in sauce

Foods containing eggs

Foods containing egg yolk, egg white and lecithin should be avoided. The following may contain eggs:

baked foods – cakes, biscuits, pastry and batter
egg noodles and pasta
lemon curd
malted milk drinks, e.g. Bournvita
mayonnaise
puddings and mixes
soups

Foods containing wheat

Wheat is present in the products listed below. Check all labels on manufactured foods. If wheat, wheat starch, edible starch, modified starch, cereal filler, cereal binder or cereal protein appear in the ingredients do not use that product. Foods marked with an asterisk may or may not contain wheat.

Beverages
cocoa,* drinking chocolate,* coffee essence,* milk shake flavourings,* Horlicks, Ovaltine*

Biscuits
homemade and bought

Bread
including white, wholemeal, wholewheat, granary breads, rye bread,* slimming bread

Breakfast cereals
e.g. Shredded Wheat, Puffed Wheat, All-Bran, Weetabix, Shreddies, muesli,* baby cereals*

Cakes
including homemade and bought cakes, cake mixes and scones

Dairy products and fats
cheese spreads,* processed cheese,* packet suet*

Fish
tinned,* fish paste,* fish cooked in batter, breadcrumbs or a sauce

Flours and cereals
ordinary wheat flours, bran, wheatgerm, semolina, pasta, noodles, couscous

Fruit
pie fillings*

Meat
tinned,* ready meals,* pies, sausage rolls, meat paste,* pâté,* sausages*

Pastry
homemade, bought, mixes and frozen

Puddings
packet puddings, dessert mixes,* ice-cream,* mousses,* custard powder*

Vegetables
tinned in sauces, e.g. baked beans,* tinned vegetable salad,* instant potato powder*

Miscellaneous
stuffings, savoury spreads,* mayonnaise,* curry powder,* mustard,* chutney,* mincemeat,* peanut butter,* lemon curd,* sweets and chocolates,* baking powder,* gravy

browning,* stock cubes,* soy sauce,* pepper compounds, packet seasonings

Foods containing yeast

The following products can, and frequently do, contain yeast in one form or another:

bread – any kind of bread, except soda bread

bread sauce, bread pudding, stuffings made with bread-crumbs, breadcrumb coatings on, e.g. fish fingers, fish cakes, potato croquettes

buns made with yeast, e.g. teacakes, rolls, crumpets, doughnuts

cheese, buttermilk, soured cream, synthetic cream

cream crackers, Twiglets

fermented beverages, e.g. wine, beer, cider

fruit juice (home squeezed citrus fruits are yeast-free)

yeast extract, Bovril, most stock cubes and gravy browning, tinned and packet soups

grapes, sultanas, currants, plums, dates, prunes and products containing these, e.g. fruit cake, mincemeat, muesli, raisin bran

malted milk drinks, e.g. Ovaltine, Horlicks

meat products containing bread, e.g. sausages, meat loaf, beefburgers

overripe fruit

pizza

puddings made with bread, e.g. apple charlotte, summer pudding

vinegar and pickled foods, e.g. pickled onions, pickled beetroot, sauces containing vinegar, e.g. tomato ketchup, salad dressing, mayonnaise

vitamin products – most B vitamin products contain yeast

Foods containing corn

The products listed below can, and frequently do, contain corn in one form or another, as cornstarch, oil, syrup or cornmeal. Modified starch, edible starch, food starch, maize oil, glucose syrup, vegetable oil and dextrose may also be derived from corn. Always check the label on manufactured products. Products marked with an asterisk may or may not contain corn.

baking mixtures for cakes and biscuits*
baking powders*
bleached white flour
bottle sauces – many contain food starch or syrup*
cakes and biscuits*
canned foods, e.g. soups, puddings, baked beans*
cornflakes
cornflour
custard powder
gravy browning
ices, ice-creams*
instant puddings*
instant teas, e.g. lemon tea mix contains dextrose
jams, jellies*
margarine and vegetable oils containing corn oil
peanut butter*
polenta
popcorn
salad dressings*
sweets – may be sweetened with corn syrup, e.g. sherbets,
    marshmallows
tortillas

Appendix B

Artificial colouring-, preservative- and salicylate-free diet

'E' numbers describe both natural and artificial colours and preservatives. It is not necessary to avoid all 'E' numbers. Check the ingredients listed on all processed and convenience foods, i.e. tins, packets, jars, bottled and ready-to-eat meals, for the following additives:

Artificial colours

Azo dyes are chemicals containing nitrogen and used as colourings in food, drinks and cosmetics. They may aggravate your condition so it is important that you avoid the following additives:

E102	tartrazine	E128	red 2G
E104	quinoline yellow	E131	patent blue carmine
E107	yellow 2G	E132	indigo
E110	sunset yellow	E133	brilliant blue FCF
E122	carmoisine	E151	black PN
E123	amaranth	E154	brown FK
E124	ponceau 4R	E155	chocolate brown HT
E127	erythrosine	E180	pigment rubine

Some foods may be coloured with natural colourings which can be included in your diet, such as E101 (riboflavin) and E160(a) (alpha carotene).

Artificial preservatives

Benzoates and sulphates are two main groups of preservatives added to certain foods by manufacturers. It is important to exclude from your diet E210–E219 (benzoates) and E220–E227 (sulphates). Also exclude the antioxidants E320 BHA and E321 BHT.

Try to include as many fresh foods as possible in your diet.

Salicylates

Salicylates are found in medicines containing aspirin, salicylate or salicylic acid. Your pharmacist will advise you about any medicines you buy. They are also found naturally in certain foods.

Foods high in salicylates are:

Berries such as blackberries, blueberries and raspberries; apples, oranges, pineapple, plums and rhubarb; dried fruit and grapes
Tomatoes, gherkins and cucumbers
All nuts, especially peanuts and almonds
Tea, coffee, wine, sherry, beer and cider
Liquorice, Marmite, curry powder, herbs and spices, Worcester sauce, white vinegar

Foods for an artificial colouring-, preservative- and salicylate-free diet

It is important to check all labels carefully, because ingredients of manufactured foods are liable to change.

	Not allowed	Allowed
Breads and cereals	Brown or white bread	100% wholemeal bread, oats, rye, corn, rice; breakfast cereals free from colours and preservatives, e.g. Shredded Wheat, Weetabix

	Not allowed	*Allowed*
Crispbread		Wheat and rye based
Pasta	Caution: some pastas contain colouring, check contents on packet	Spaghetti, macaroni, vermicelli, etc.
Cakes and biscuits	Commercially prepared varieties, including special cake mixes	Home-made varieties using permitted ingredients
Vegetables	Canned and commercially bottled; tomatoes, gherkins, cucumbers	Fresh, frozen, dried, domestically bottled
Fruit	Berries, apples, oranges, pineapple, plums, rhubarb, grapes, dried fruit Caution: check frozen fruit and fruit juices	Fresh, frozen and bottled
Milk	Flavoured milk	Fresh, long-life (UHT), sterilized, skimmed, dried milk powder
Cream	Artificial creams	Fresh
Yoghurt	Coloured or flavoured yoghurt	Natural yoghurt
Meat and fish	Cured and pre-cooked meats, smoked fish, meat and fish products	Fresh meat and fish
Beverages	Squashes, beer, cider, wine, tea, coffee, fruit juices (see above)	Water, fruit and herbal teas

Useful addresses

Useful websites
www.irritablebowelsyndrome.co.uk
www.crohns.org.uk

Associations
Migraine Action Associaton
Unit 6
Oakley Hay Lodge Business Park
Great Folds Road
Great Oakley
Northants NN18 9AS
Tel: Ms Helen Sinclair 01536 461333
E-mail: info@migraine.org.uk
Website: www.migraine.org.uk

National Eczema Society
Hill House
Highgate Hill
London N19 5NA
Office Tel: 020 7281 3553
Helpline: 0870 241 3604
Website: www.eczema.org

Coeliac Society
PO Box 220
High Wycombe HP11 2HY
Tel: 01494 437278
Website: www.coeliac.co.uk

National Association for Colitis and Crohn's Disease (NACC)
4 Beaumont House
Sutton Road
St Albans
Herts AL1 5HH
Support line: 0845 130 3344
Website: www.nacc.org.uk

The Arthritis Research Campaign
PO Box 177
Chesterfield
Derbyshire S41 7TQ
Tel: 0870 850 5000
Website: www.arc.org.uk

Supermarket nutrition services

The following services provide information on their products,
i.e. milk-free, gluten-free etc.

Asda
Customer Services
Asda house
Great Wilson St
Leeds LS11 5AD
Tel: 0500 100055
Website: www.asda.co.uk

CO-OP
Customer Services
Freepost MR9 473
Manchester M4 8BA
Tel: 08000 686727
Website: www.co-op.co.uk

Marks and Spencer
Retail Customer Services
Chester Business Park
Wrexham Road
Chester CH14 9GA
Tel: 0845 302 1234
Website: www.marksandspencer.com

Morrisons
Customer Services Department
Parry Lane
Bradford BD4 8TD
Tel: 01274 356000
Website: www.morrisons.co.uk

Sainsbury
33 Holborn
London EC1N 2HT
Tel: 0800 636 262
Website: www.sainsbury.co.uk

Somerfield
Customer Relations
Somerfield House
Whitchurch Lane
Bristol BS14 0TJ
Tel: 01179 359359
Website: www.somerfield.co.uk

Tesco
Tesco Customer Service Centre
Tesco House
Delamare Road
Cheshunt
Herts EN8 9SL
Tel: 0800 505 555
Website: www.tesco.com

Waitrose
Nutrition Advice Service
Doncastle Road
Bracknell
Berks RG12 8YA
Tel: 0800 188 884
Website: www.waitrose.com

Manufacturers supplying special dietary products

There are a number of companies manufacturing dietary foods
that may be suitable for multiple exclusion diets such as
gluten-, milk- and egg-free. Some of the main suppliers are
listed below. These usually have a mail order service and their
products may be found in health food shops or supermarkets.

Barbara's Kitchen Ltd
Unit 16
Ely Valley Business Park (East)
Pontyclun
South Wales CF72 9ES

D and D Chocolates
Centenary Business Centre
Attleborough Industrial Estate
Nuneaton CV11 6RY

General Dietary Ltd
PO Box 38
Kingston upon Thames
Surrey KT2 7YP
Tel: 020 8336 2323
(Brand name: *Ener-G*)

Gluten Free Foods Ltd
Unit 270
Centennial Park
Centennial Ave
Elstree
Borehamwood
Herts WD6 3SS
Tel: 020 8953 4444
Website: www.glutenfree-foods.co.uk
(Brand names: *Glutano* and *Barkat*)

Lifestyle Healthcare Ltd
Centenary Business Park
Henley-on-Thames RG9 1DS
Tel: 01491 570000
Website: www.gfdiet.com
(Brand names: *Lifestyle, Allergycare* and *Ultra*)

Nutricia Dietary Care Ltd
Newmarket Avenue
Whitehorse Business Park
Trowbridge
Wilts BA14 0XQ
Tel: 01225 711801
Orders: 0870 241 5954
Website: www.glutafin.co.uk
(Brand names: *Glutafin* and *Trufree*)

Scientific Hospital Supplies
100 Wavertree Boulevard
Liverpool L7 9BT
Tel: 0151 228 8161
Websites: www.shsweb.co.uk or www.juvela.co.uk
(Brand name: *Juvela*)

Community Foods
Micross
Brent Terrace
Brent Cross
London NW2 1LT
Tel: 020 8450 9411
Website: www.communityfoods.co.uk
(Brand name: *Orgran*)

Nutrition Point Ltd
13 Taurus Park
Westbrook
Warrington WA5 7ZT
Tel: 07041 544044
Website: www.nutritionpoint.co.uk
(Brand names: *Dietary specials* and *Schar*)

Doves Farm
Salisbury Road
Hungerford
Berks RG17 0RF
Tel: 01488 684 880
Website: www.dovesfarm.co.uk

Index

Recipes suitable for special diets are indicated as explained on page 76: exclusion (*), milk-free (M), LOFFLEX (L), wheat-free (W), egg-free (E). Children's recipes are indicated by C.